LESSONS
FROM THE
HEART

*Individualizing Physical Education
With Heart Rate Monitors*

Beth Kirkpatrick
NASPE Teacher of the Year
Emens Distinguished Professor, Ball State University

Burton H. Birnbaum
Vice Chairman, Polar Electro, Inc.

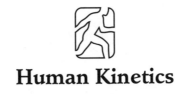

Human Kinetics

Library of Congress Cataloging-in-Publication Data

Kirkpatrick, Beth, 1931-
    Lessons from the heart : individualizing physical education with
heart rate monitors / Beth Kirkpatrick, Burton H. Birnbaum.
        p.   cm.
    Includes bibliographical references (p.   ) and index.
    ISBN 0-88011-764-8 (alk. paper)
    1. Physical education and training.   2. Heart rate monitoring.
3. Exercise--Physiological aspects.   4. Individualized instruction.
5. Lesson planning.   I. Birnbaum, Burton H., 1942-   . II. Title.
GV362.K47   1997
613.7'04--dc21   96-53062
                                                                CIP

ISBN: 0-88011-764-8

Acquisitions Editor: Scott Wikgren; **Developmental Editor:** Julie Rhoda; **Assistant Editor:** Sandra Merz Bott; **Editorial Assistant:** Jennifer Jeanne Hemphill; **Copyeditor:** Bonnie Pettifor; **Proofreader:** Erin Cler; **Graphic Designer:** Judy Henderson; **Graphic Artist:** Yvonne Winsor; **Photo Editor:** Boyd LaFoon; **Cover Designer:** Jack Davis; **Photographer (cover):** Michael Moffett; **Cover Models:** Teacher—Lynne Srull, Kids—Marquis Johnson and Kari Reineke; **Illustrator:** Sara Giroux Wolfsmith, Gerald Barrett; **Printer:** Versa Press; Interior photos on pp. 7, 23, and 99 courtesy of Polar Electro, Inc.

A special thanks to all the children and parents who participated in the photo shoots.

Printed in the United States of America   10 9 8 7 6 5 4 3

Human Kinetics
Web site: www.humankinetics.com

United States: Human Kinetics, P.O. Box 5076, Champaign, IL 61825-5076
800-747-4457
e-mail: humank@hkusa.com

Canada: Human Kinetics, 475 Devonshire Road, Unit 100, Windsor, ON N8Y 2L5
800-465-7301 (in Canada only)
e-mail: humank@hkcanada.com

Europe: Human Kinetics, P.O. Box IW14, Leeds LS16 6TR, United Kingdom
+44 (0)113-278 1708
e-mail: humank@hkeurope.com

Australia: Human Kinetics, 57A Price Avenue, Lower Mitcham, South Australia 5062
(08) 82771555
e-mail: liahka@senet.com.au

New Zealand: Human Kinetics, P.O. Box 105-231, Auckland Central
09-309-1890
e-mail: humank@hknewz.com

Contents

Chapter 6 Advanced Lesson Plans   79

Chapter 7 Heart Rate Sports: Games for All Ages   99

Preface

We have written *Lessons From the Heart* with several thoughts in mind. First, no greater tool for use in the field of physical education has been invented than the heart rate monitor. It's like looking through a window into the heart. Indeed, a heart rate monitor gives your students the information they need to determine for themselves when to increase or decrease exercise intensity, which is a function of heart rate. Thus, this technology makes it possible for you to make your students accountable for their individual efforts. In turn, you can be accountable to your students, their parents, and your school's administration because you have concrete, objective data to support the grades you give.

We speak from experience. A seasoned physical educator, Beth has reviewed over 15,000 heart rate printouts from the students of her physical education classes in Vinton, Iowa. She has downloaded information collected during a wide variety of activities, which have even included students giving speeches! Using the Polar Vantage XL Heart Rate Monitor, she has administered the traditional mile-run cardiovascular test to each of her students since 1982, watching for consistent effort through heart rate comparisons of the fall and the spring tests. The documentation, which only this technology can provide, has given her great peace of mind, both knowing that she is giving objective credit as she rewards students for doing their personal bests, and that she

is providing for safety through applying technology in physical education by not pushing students beyond their physical capabilities.

Burt, who holds master's degrees in both engineering and business, designed his first pulsemeter over 20 years ago. As early as 1977 he was involved in experimental programs for motivating obese students to partake in physical activity that brought their heart rate into a predetermined zone. Burt's technical and business acumen bring a new dimension to the physical education applications of technology. As a parent of an elementary school teacher and a grandparent, he is very much interested and involved in ensuring that physical education results in a life-long, active, healthy lifestyle.

But perhaps the greatest benefit of this technology has been to be able to look into the hearts of our students, thereby earning their trust. We, as their teachers, are giving them the chance to exercise according to their individual levels of fitness. By allowing them the chance to move to the beat of their own hearts, we give them the gifts from the heart of independence, success no matter what the student's ability, and personal responsibility for fitness. Indeed, heart rate monitors take your curriculum beyond physical fitness as they help you teach valuable life skills. You don't have to guess what is right for students, either. Teach through science and document what is going on in your classes, student by student.

As you plan your overall curriculum and specific lessons, it is important to recognize that heart rate is very individual: No two people will ever have the same heart rate response to every lesson. Use heart rate monitors to measure individual responses, allowing students to vary intensity accordingly, to obtain maximum benefits in complete safety. Exercise-induced asthmatic children, for example, can be physically active knowing that the heart rate monitor will warn them if their heart rates are going too high.

Specifically, we have designed these lessons to give you ideas for how to use the information that the heart rate monitor can provide across the curriculum from the youngest to the oldest students, from elementary school through college and beyond, in physical education as well as athletics. Through using heart rate monitors, we are able to meet the needs of such a wide range of students because the heart rate reflects more than cardiovascular fitness. For example, heart rate can tell us how hard we are working, the level of stress in our lives, the effects of heat and cold on the body, the need to control anger and hostility, if drug abuse is occurring, and the body's day-to-day responses to exercise.

The more we discovered the information heart rate can reflect, the more we recognized the importance of getting this information to as many educators as possible. Certainly, no other teaching tool combines authentic assessment, life skills lessons, and accountability into one compete and easy-to-apply package. We believe that once you embark on the exciting adventure of the heart rate monitor, you will discover even more applications of this technology. In fact, we are counting on you to bring new ideas to this fascinating world. Let us know how you are applying these lessons as well as about the lessons you have created yourself by writing to the attention of Burt Birnbaum at Polar Electro, Inc., 99 Seaview Blvd., Port Washington, NY 11050. We would love to add your "lessons from the heart" to the next edition.

Introduction

Videos, computer games, and parents failing to encourage children to be physically active are just a few of the reasons today's children are growing up inactive. Years ago, we could take for granted that children would engage in fun physical activity. But nowadays, encouraging children to partake in physical activity falls to the schools, and in particular to physical education departments. Children's lack of physical activity has declined so far that in 1995 the Surgeon General found it necessary to report the effects of inactivity on children's health. (The only other time that a Surgeon General has felt so strongly about an issue to write a report was regarding smoking.) Furthermore, the importance of young people exercising can be seen in a recent British study, which found that "people who exercise regularly in their youth are more likely to continue or to resume exercise in later years." For example, 25 percent of the youth who were active when they were 14 to 19 years old were very active as adults compared to 2 percent of the sedentary adolescents becoming active adults (The Sports Council 1992).

The purpose of *Lessons From the Heart* is to present ideas to you, the educator, that not only motivate children to participate in aerobic exercise but also to educate both you and your students alike as to the potential for authentically assessing fitness that heart rate monitors provide.

Moreover, using heart rate monitors makes aerobic exercise safer and more productive by helping you and your students individualize participation in physical activity. A student utilizing a heart rate monitor can guide himself to his individual exercise level. Instead of comparing himself to others, he may now concentrate on competing against his previous efforts. In this way, it is possible to give every student the experience of success by pointing out that he can exercise as efficiently as anyone else. When you reward effort instead of elite performance, the self-esteem of the unfit student rises dramatically as he performs physical activity within his target heart rate zone, at the same level of effort as his peers. All students learn that the individual's heart rate, not competition, is the common goal.

But this book isn't only about heart rates and technology! It's about teaching and supporting a lifestyle that includes regular physical activity. And you can plant the seed in the primary grades that will grow into the flower of a lifestyle of fitness. In fact, the sooner children become "hooked" on physical activity, the better. Later in the upper grades of elementary school, they may become prejudiced against physical activity as their bodies begin to undergo a series of changes that may be embarrassing to them, making it more difficult for them to have positive exercise experiences.

Using heart rate monitors in physical education facilitates an interesting opportunity for monitoring both the heart and well-being. As the teaching tool of the 21st century, the heart rate monitor enhances interdisciplinary technological instruction while allowing for a more objective estimation of a student's effort and individual progress, instead of relying on how an individual's performance compares to others' performances. Moreover, heart rate monitors provide both you and your students with immediate feedback on the efficiency of various physical activities in a variety of sports, helping students learn to exercise more efficiently. Apply this valuable data when planning physical education lessons to tailor your curriculum to your students' needs.

This book presents only a sampling of the possibilities that exist for using heart rate monitors in the teaching-learning process. Chapter 1 includes basic information about the function of the heart and the whys and hows of measuring heart rates. Chapter 2 provides some suggested class procedures and ideas for easily distributing heart rate monitors during class time and tracking each student's fitness via heart rate throughout the school term. Chapter 3 then gets you started on heart rate calculation and analysis with three assessment lessons using heart rate monitors: finding your students' maximum and resting heart rates and completing the mile-run test.

Chapters 4, 5, and 6 include 30 sample lesson plans for the beginner, intermediate, and advanced heart rate monitor users, students in kindergarten through high school. Along with a stated goal, key concepts, equipment needed, and activity procedures, each lesson includes teaching tips as well as note sections for you to write your own lesson observations, ideas, or modifications. Chapter 7 includes five additional lessons using heart rate monitors within sports games. But beyond providing you with basic information and sample lessons, we hope that *Lessons From the Heart* helps you develop an interdisci-

plinary approach to using technology to advocate a healthy lifestyle. We believe that this is the path to higher levels of learning and to the next century.

So work with your colleagues to integrate heart rate data across the curriculum. For example, the heart rate data gathered during a lesson in physical education may be used for demonstrating physiology in biology lessons: the functioning of the heart and the circulatory system as well as of hormones and nerves. Or in an information technology or a language arts lesson, students may write a report on the basis of a heart rate curve printout of data collected throughout an entire day, pondering the reasons for changes in heart rate and its effect on fitness.

In this age of authentic assessment, heart rate monitors are a must. To help you see how they can help you teach, comply with, and assess achievement against the national standards, we have addressed this issue in relation to the NASPE Content Standards for Physical Education in appendix B. In summary, heart rate monitors provide the concrete, objective data for measuring effort, creating for the first time true accountability in physical education. Specifically, you can download heart rate data to a computer, then print it out. Place the printouts in students' portfolios for accurate, ongoing documentation. Give students and parents copies, teaching them how to interpret the information so that families can address fitness in specific ways. Furthermore, heart rate monitors help students enjoy physical activity more—not because they view them as technological toys, but because they feel empowered to function *and achieve* at their own ability levels. Thus, we encourage you to empower both yourself and your students with this authentic assessment tool as you strive to learn these lessons for the heart.

The Heart and Heart Rate

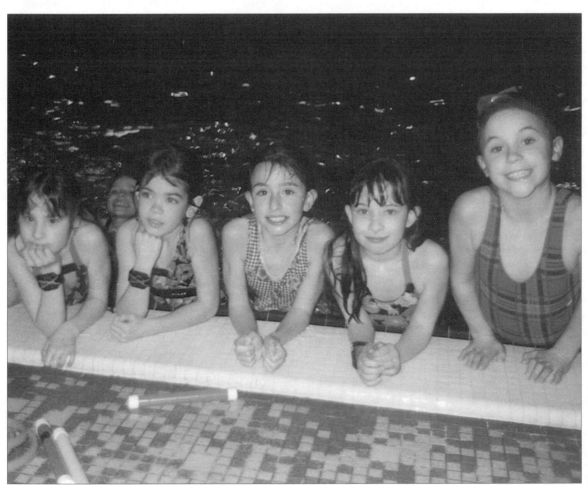

Photo courtesy of Arleen Corson

Accurate assessment of the heart rate response to exercise represents the simplest and most valuable piece of information available to students and teachers alike. The rate that the heart is beating is a reliable and effective measure of the physiological changes occurring within the exerciser. Thus, knowing the age of the student and assuming good health, you can determine a safe optimum range for exercise heart rate.

Structure and Function of the Heart

The heart is the most vital organ of your body, the engine that, when contracting, pumps blood to the lungs and to the trunk and lower extremities. The heart is located under your chest bone, partly in the upper left quadrant, but nearly in the center of your chest.

The heart is a muscle the size of your fist. The heart of any average size adult weighs less than half a kilogram (1.1 pounds). If you regularly perform physical exercise that improves your stamina, in the long run, your heart—like any muscle within the body—may grow larger. During maximum performance, the heart of a person with average fitness is capable of flowing more strongly than a kitchen tap running at full force.

The heart muscle consists of two pumps, both of which have two chambers separated by valves (figure 1.1). Carbon-dioxide-laden blood travels through veins from all parts of the body to the right half of the heart muscle, called the right atrium. From the right atrium, the heart pumps the blood to a second chamber, called the right ventricle, which in turn pumps the blood to the lungs. In the lungs, the blood releases its stored carbon dioxide gases and absorbs atmospheric oxygen.

Oxygen-rich blood flows from the lungs to a chamber on the left side of the heart, called the left atrium, and from there to the left ventricle, from which the heart pumps it to the aorta and finally to the body through the arteries.

The heart functions in two phases: contraction (systole) and rest (diastole). When the heart contracts and blood flows to the rest of the body, it

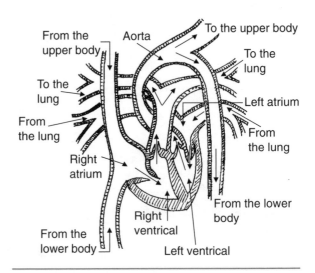

Figure 1.1 *The structure of the heart.*

does so at a certain amount of pressure. When the heart muscle is at rest, the pressure in the vessels decreases. These two pressures, the higher pressure at contraction (systolic pressure) and the lower pressure at rest (diastolic pressure) are the two numbers found when your blood pressure is measured. We call the heart muscle's contractions heartbeats, generally measuring them in beats per minute.

Your heart rate, like your blood pressure, is generally controlled involuntarily by a natural pacemaker located in your heart's upper right atrium. This pacemaker, the sinus, is a bundle of specialized muscle tissues that receives regulating messages from your brain. If your cells need more oxygen, the brain automatically accelerates the heart's pumping activity, increasing blood flow.

The complete heartbeat sequence is similar to a musical rhythm, consisting of a sequence of electrical activities occurring in a specific set of patterns. The sequence of events starts with the valves between the chambers opening and closing, continues as the heart muscle contracts, and finishes during the postcontraction relaxation, or pause. Throughout the contraction phase, the heart pumps blood out. The relaxation phase of the rhythm allows time for blood to refill the chambers. An ECG can record this information. Cardiologists and exercise scientists use ECGs to obtain and study accurate heart rate information. Through ECGs, experts can discover any abnormalities in the functioning of the heart. Figure 1.2 presents part of a sample ECG.

Heartbeat Intervals (in seconds)

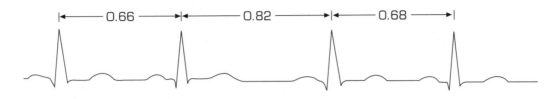

Figure 1.2 *Part of a sample ECG.*

Specifically, an ECG is a grahic presentation of a sequence of electrical events in the heart that follow each other in a certain rhythmic pattern. An ECG can register the cardiac rhythm either on chart paper or on the oscilloscope display by using two or more electrodes attached to the chest and to the measuring device. The electrodes measure the electrical activity going through the heart. Similarly, the chest transmitters of the better heart rate monitors accurately determine when the heart beats and, without wires, transmit the pulse reading to the wristwatch receiver.

Factors Affecting Heart Function

The heart regulates its functions automatically, but several factors can affect its contraction. Let's examine brief descriptions of some of these factors that affect the heart rate in various situations.

Body Position

Heart rate is lowest in the supine position and highest when standing. The more the muscles work, the more they require oxygen-rich blood, therefore, the higher the heart rate.

Fitness

Fit persons have a lower working and resting heart rate. The resting heart rate of a fit person can be less than 40 beats per minute, whereas an untrained person in poor condition may have a resting heart rate of over 100 beats per minute.

Endurance training strengthens the heart and improves the functioning of the circulatory system, for example, by enlarging the volume of the left chamber, which allows the heart to pump more blood with one contraction, and thus leads to a lowered resting heart rate. The more fit the person is, the more blood the heart is able to pump every time it beats and the more slowly the heart beats to perform the same workload.

Age

The following target range chart indicates how optimum heart rates change as a function of age (figure 1.3).

Gender

Typically, adult women have a heart rate five to seven beats per minute (bpm) higher than that of males. This is because they have proportionately smaller hearts and other muscles.

Mood

Various situations that excite your mind, such as stage fright or an unpleasant experience, can make your heart rate rise. Prolonged periods of stress increase heart rate as well. Conversely, when you are relaxed, inhaling and exhaling in a peaceful manner, and thinking about something pleasant, your heart rate lowers.

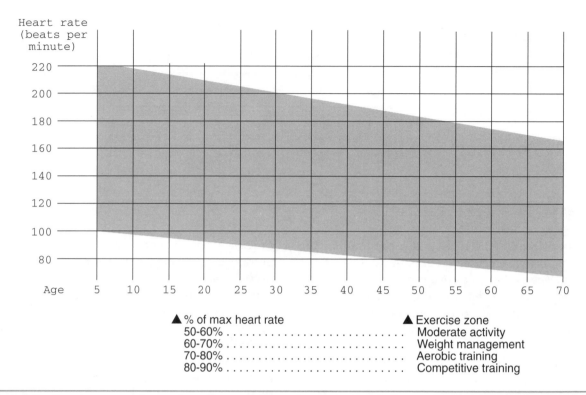

Figure 1.3   Target zone exercise produces the maximum cardiovascular benefit for your heart and helps achieve your fitness goals effectively.

Temperature

Heart rate and changes in your body's temperature are directly related: the higher the temperature, the higher your heart rate.

Stimulants

Smoking and caffeinated beverages such as coffee, tea, and cola drinks increase heart rate. The effect of caffeinated products on heart rate is minor, but smoking may increase resting heart rate temporarily by more than 10 beats per minute. At any given time, a smoker's resting heart rate is generally higher than that of a nonsmoker because the blood's capacity to transport oxygen is weaker.

Depressants

A small amount of alcohol usually relaxes and thus lowers the heart rate. Exercising when un-

der the influence of alcohol is not healthy as it leads to fatigue much faster than in a person not under the influence, increases heart rate, and predisposes the person to accidents.

Surgeon General's Report

The importance of participating in regular physical activity and the value of good physical education programs in schools is readily addressed in the Surgeon General's *Report on Physical Activity and Health*, drafted in 1995, which states, "The Surgeon General has determined that lack of physical activity is detrimental to your health" (U.S. Department of Health and Human Services 1996). The Surgeon General has only published one other report addressing a major public health concern: that of smoking.

The following are among the report's major findings:

- People who are usually inactive can improve their health and well-being by becoming even moderately active on a regular basis.
- Physical activity need not be strenuous to achieve health benefits.
- A person can achieve greater health benefits by increasing the amount (duration, frequency, or intensity) of physical activity.

Why Monitor Heart Rate?

It's not surprising that the Surgeon General of the United States has determined that lack of physical activity is detrimental to your health. But how do we as individuals determine how much physical activity is enough to achieve good health? The simplest means of determining how much is to listen to your own body; listen to your heart—learn how fast it is beating. Physicians have asserted that 20 minutes of "good" cardiovascular exercise a minimum of three times a week is essential to good health. "Good" cardiovascular exercise depends on keeping your heart rate in the target zone for your age as shown in figure 1.3.

Letting your heart rate guide your exercise intensity to obtain optimum benefits is analogous to using the cruise control function on your car, which automatically increases and decreases gas flow as a function of speed. The purpose of cruise control is to enable us to get from point A to point B as fast as possible (benefit) without getting a ticket (safety). The heart rate monitor allows you to exercise at a constant heart rate (varying exercise intensity is analogous to varying the pressure on the gas pedal) to obtain your maximum health benefits in complete safety.

Measuring Heart Rate

You can measure the workload of the heart either manually by feeling your pulse at specific checkpoints on your body or electronically by using a heart rate monitor.

Palpation Method

In the manual, or palpation, measurement, you measure the number of beats at the arteries on your wrist, for example, for a period of 15 seconds (figure 1.4). To measure manually, press the forefinger and the middle finger lightly on the wrist's inner side under the thumb. Start counting from 0, 1, 2, 3, and so on, and then multiply the result of the calculation by four.

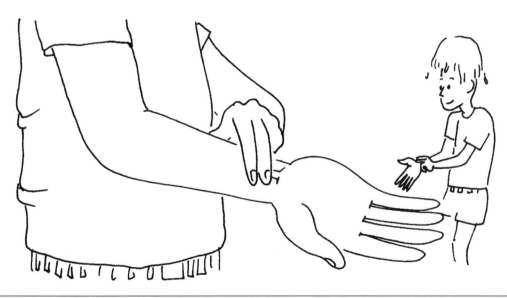

Figure 1.4   In the palpation method, feel for your pulse at your wrist with your forefinger and middle finger. Count the number of heartbeats for 15 seconds and multiply by four.

Unfortunately, measuring the pulse by this method during physical exercise is inaccurate as it is most often done only after the exercise, and thus easily leads to timing and calculation problems. Furthermore, the higher the heart rate, the greater the potential error, and typically the figure derived by feeling the pulse is lower than in reality. Regardless of whether you count for 15 seconds or a full minute, errors as high as plus or minus 15 beats per minute on exercise heart rate are typical.

Electronic Measurement

There are two main types of electronic meters: pulsemeters and ECG-based meters. The typical pulsemeter measures the blood flow rate in the finger or earlobe by shining light into the skin and sensing changes in light density in the photoelectric sensor; the pulsemeter then calculates and displays the rate in bpm. Heart rate monitors measure the electrical activity of the heart through the electrodes worn on the chest and count the number of signals that tell the heart to beat. Polar heart rate monitors, which are ECG accurate and easy to use, transmit heart rate telemetrically (without wires) to a wristwatch-type receiver.

The difference between the ECG and the heart rate monitor is fairly simple: An ECG gives a picture of the complete cardiac rhythm while the heart rate monitor only measures one part of the cardiac rhythm—the number of times your heart beats. The Polar heart rate monitor consists of three parts: a lightweight transmitter, which you wear on your chest, an elastic strap for attaching the transmitter to the skin, and a receiver, which you can wear on your wrist. The Polar transmitter is attached to your chest with an elastic strap. The length of the strap is adjustable to fit different sizes of chests. The transmitter contains two electrodes that sense from the skin the electric signals coming from the beating heart. The transmitter sends the heartbeat to the wrist receiver with the help of an electromagnetic field but without wires. The current heart rate (beats per minute) is visible on the receiver's display at any time.

In the classroom, heart rate monitors permit students to exercise at ideal intensity to attain, record, and maintain accountability to both themselves and the teacher while engaging in "good" cardiovascular exercise. Students, through heart rate monitoring, can now let their bodies guide themselves (biofeedback) to achieve maximum benefits for minimum efforts—all while having fun.

CHAPTER

2

Using Heart Rate Monitors in Class

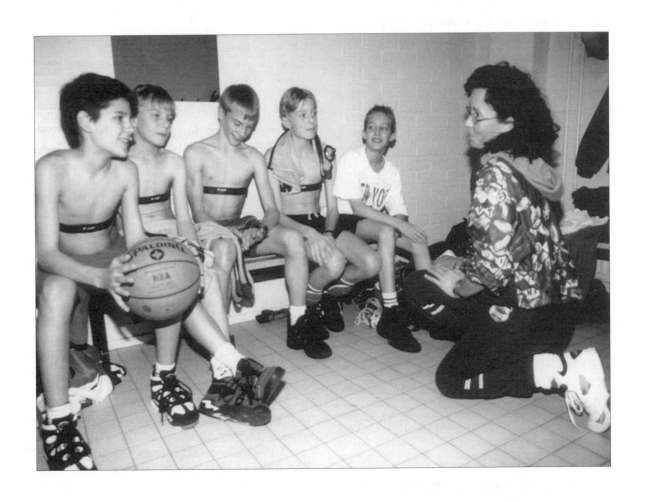

As we mentioned in chapter 1, fitness increases the heart's efficiency, resulting in a healthier body, a body that permits you to do more without tiring, a body you can be proud of. A few of the changes that occur as we get more and more fit include the following.

Efficiency of Exercise

Physiological Changes

The heart muscle becomes stronger.

The heart's internal circulation improves.

The resting heart rate lowers.

The heart's stroke volume (specifically due to endurance training) and the volume per minute increases.

The heart's contraction capacity improves.

The muscles' capacity to use oxygen improves.

The body's oxygen intake capacity improves.

The blood's capacity to transport oxygen improves because the number of red blood corpuscles increases.

Physiological Effects of Exercise on the Human Body That May Prevent Health Problems

The blood's triglyceride content decreases.

The amount of HDL cholesterol (the good cholesterol) increases.

Control of the metabolism of sugars improves (more stable blood sugar concentration; lowered risk of maturity-onset diabetes).

Secretion of adrenal hormones (stress hormones) decreases with regular exercise.

Diastolic blood pressure lowers.

Subcutaneous body fat decreases (person loses body fat).

Other Effects

The level of muscular strength is preserved or improves.

The bones become stronger.

The working capacity of joints is preserved or improves.

Stress decreases and relaxation increases.

Self-confidence improves.

Social and emotional health improves.

Exerciser feels refreshed.

Using a heart rate monitor while exercising helps us to achieve these positive benefits, starting us on the road to a healthy lifestyle.

Monitoring Effort

The best means for monitoring physical strain, or effort, is to measure heart rate. The higher the heart rate, the more strenuous we can say the exercises are for a particular person. Heart rate is a useful property to measure during and after the exercise since it gives you individual feedback on your performance. Indeed, each person reacts to physical strain individually, depending on the size of the heart, fitness level, skills, and daily changes of mood. The heart rate of a fit person recovers after exercise back to the resting rate faster than that of a person in poor condition.

Measuring heart rates with a heart rate monitor encourages each student to exercise at a sufficiently strenuous level. The self-esteem of students at lower fitness levels than their peers, especially those who typically avoid exercise, increases dramatically as they take part in physical activity and achieve grades proportional to their documented efforts. In other words, using a heart rate monitor allows you to base grades on level of effort and degree of improvement, rather than on absolute achievement—very encouraging to less fit students and motivating to students at all fitness levels.

Maximum and Resting Heart Rates

Your maximum heart rate represents your heart's highest possible beating density, or your heart rate in a situation when it no longer rises even if the strain still does. Table 2.1 shows referential values for maximum heart rates in various age groups. Highly reputable studies have also been made of children's maximum heart rates. In a British study (Armstrong 1991) on students 11 to 16 years of age, the average maximum heart rates were:

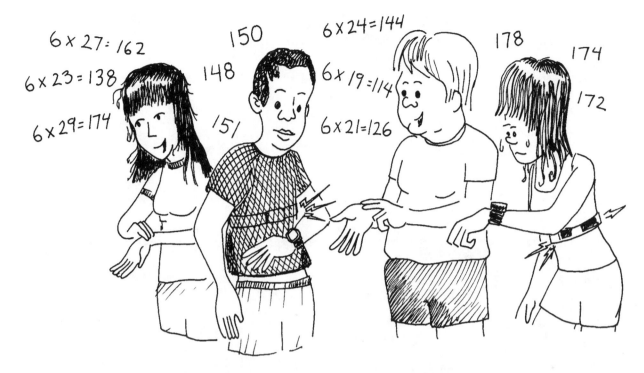

- boys (113 informants) 200 beats per minute (plus or minus eight beats), and
- girls (107 informants) 201 beats per minute (plus or minus eight beats).

The results show the variation in the maximum heart rates of children. On the basis of this research, we may conclude that we can apply the referential values of maximum heart rates shown in table 2.1 to children when calculating children's target heart rate zones.

In addition to maximum heart rate, another essential number is the resting heart rate, or the lowest number of beats per minute your heart contracts at rest. The best time to measure the resting heart rate is when you wake up in the morning, while still lying peacefully in bed before you lift your head from the pillow. You can most accurately define your resting heart rate, for example, by measuring the heart rate in this way for a sequence of six days, then calculating the average of those values (see chapter 3, lesson 1).

Target Heart Rate Zones

A target heart rate zone is the heart rate zone within which the heart should beat to achieve the desired physiological benefits. The most common way to calculate your target heart rate zone is by finding percentages of your maximum heart rate (HRmax). The appropriate target heart rate zone for physical exercise depends on what you are aiming for.

Here are examples of possible target heart rate zones:

50 to 60% HRmax = sufficiently strenuous daily exercise.

60 to 70% HRmax = efficient fat-burning zone.

70 to 80% HRmax = improvement of endurance.

80 to 100% HRmax = competitive training.

For the general activities of children a target heart rate zone of 60 to 80 percent of maximum heart rate has a positive effect on the heart and the circulatory system, without being too strenuous (see table 2.1). The level of strain is aerobic, that is, the intake of oxygen by the lungs and consumption of oxygen by the muscles are in balance.

When exercising at the anaerobic efficiency level, the consumption of oxygen is greater than its intake, which means that the muscles will have to start using their own energy resources to maintain their work. In this way, muscles are eventually filled with waste products, especially lactic acid, which makes you feel tired and which causes muscle pain.

TABLE 2.1   Average Maximum Heart Rates and the 80% and 60% Heart Rates (beats per minute, rounded to the nearest five) in childhood (Numminen and Välimäki 1995).

Age (years)	Maximum HR	80% HR	60% HR
5-8	220	175	130
9-12	210	170	125
13-16	200	160	120
17-20	200	160	120

Definitions and Concept Words

Aerobic: Exercising at a level of strain in which a person is sweating and is no more than slightly out of breath. The metabolism of muscles is receiving enough oxygen. It is generally believed that the aerobic heart rate zone is 60 to 80 percent of maximum heart rate. This level of exercise can be sustained for long periods of time.

Anaerobic: Exercising at a heavy level of strain in which a person faces fatigue quickly. The muscles have to work with insufficient oxygen supply. Typically, this exercise intensity can only be sustained for short periods (e.g., sprinting).

Anaerobic threshold: Physiological point during exercise of increasing intensity at which the blood lactate continues to accumulate such that the body is not able to synthesize it (i.e., the muscles require more oxygen than the heart via blood can transport).

Blood lactate: By-product (waste product) of the oxidation of glucose with insufficient oxygen.

Capacity per minute: The volume of blood the heart is able to pump in one minute.

Heart rate: The number of beats of the heart normally expressed as beats per minute.

Maximum heart rate: The highest number of times your heart can contract in one minute, which can be reached at maximum effort. Your maximum heart rate changes with age.

Pulse: The measure of the heart's mechanical work in the circulatory system or the number of times the heart sends blood into the expanding arteries, normally expressed as beats per minute.

Recovery heart rate: The heart rate measured at certain intervals after exercise, most often at one, three, and five minutes after completion.

Resting heart rate: The number of beats in one minute when you are at complete, uninterrupted rest. It is best taken when you first wake up in the morning before you lift your head from the pillow.

Stroke volume: The amount of blood the heart is able to pump in one contraction.

Target heart rate zone: The heart rate range within which the heart should beat to achieve the desired physiological benefits.

Polar Accurex II Heart Rate Monitor

You can have students use the Polar Accurex II Heart Rate Monitor throughout the day, as many times as needed. The information stored in the heart rate monitor is displayed immediately on conclusion of the exercise session and is automatically erased when used by the next student (figure 2.1). Thus, it is important to record information immediately before the next student uses a monitor.

The Polar Accurex II Heart Rate Monitor does the following:

- Guides the student to optimum exercise intensity through HI/LO visual and audio alarms
- Computes and displays "Quality Time," which is total exercise time in, above, and below target zone
- Computes and displays average heart rate for an entire workout
- Records 44 lap times and corresponding heart rates
- Displays recovery time information
- Resists water to 20 meters

Polar Vantage XL Heart Rate Monitor

Since the Polar Vantage XL Heart Rate Monitor stores up to eight different students, it is impor-

tant to record both the letter and file number next to student names. By carefully keeping track of results, you can use this model in back-to-back classes. At the end of the day, you should download the monitor, storing all data on disks. You can place hardcopy printouts in each child's portfolio at your convenience.

The Polar Vantage XL Heart Rate Monitor does the following:

- Guides the student to optimum exercise intensity through HI/LO visual and audio alarms
- Records the heart rate of up to eight students (in individual files) for up to eight class periods
- Includes computer interface capability, allowing you to download heart rate information to an IBM-compatible PC or Macintosh.
- Allows you to individualize each student's heart rate printout for safety and evaluation
- Resists water to 20 meters

Suggested Class Procedures

Have students wear the heart rate monitors throughout the class time. The monitors record their heart rates, and you should give students credit for using this technology correctly. The following tips will help you manage your classes:

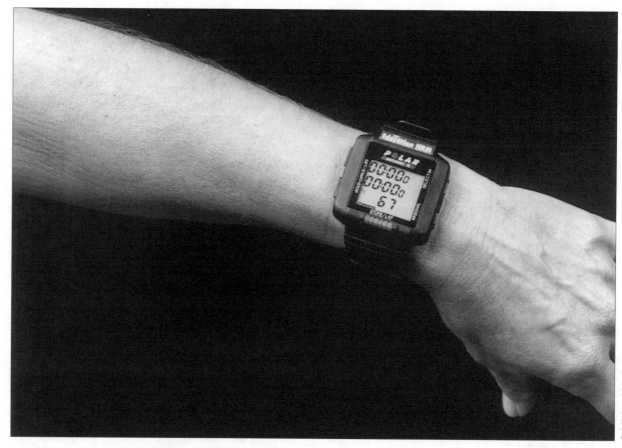

Figure 2.1   Polar Accurex II Heart Rate Monitor face.

1. Label all heart rate monitors with one letter of the alphabet for the first 26 and double letters (aa, bb, cc, and so on) thereafter.

2. Program all monitors for your students' target heart rate zones. Do so by subtracting the students' average age from 220 and multiplying this number first by .7 then by .85 (see chapter 3, lesson 2), then enter these zones into each heart rate monitor as stipulated in the owner's manual. By programming the monitors with this zone, a beep from a monitor will alert you if a student's heart rate is not in the target zone. Thus accountability for achieving proper exercise intensity is individualized in a way no other method can. Since typically all students in a class are of the same age all students will have the same target zones (unless there are medical contraindications). For athletic training, the target zone would have to be more individualized.

3. Give students the electrode chest strap before they change clothes.

4. When students are dressed and electrode chest straps are on, have students enter gym and line up behind one another to receive heart rate monitors. You may want to divide the students into groups of four to eight students and assign a squad leader for each group. Squad leaders can record which students are wearing which monitors. The same lettered heart rate monitor should be given to the same student each day.

5. After receiving a heart rate monitor, have each student immediately go to an individual exercise space, turn on the monitor, and begin the warm-up phase.

6. After all students have received their individual heart rate monitors, begin class and teach without interruption. Be sure to tell students to push the store/recall button when the aerobic segment of the class begins and to push it again when the aerobic segment of class ends. Give each student credit for following directions. Ask the students to hold their heart rates in the target zone

throughout the aerobic segment of class. If a student has too high of a heart rate, a beeper on the monitor sounds to alert her to slow down.

7. At the end of class, each student records the following information on their personalized chart. (If you have divided students into squads and assigned squad leaders, the squad leader can record this information on a chart for each student in the squad.)

Minutes in the target zone

Minutes below the target zone

Minutes above the target zone

Average heart rate throughout the class time (or from time monitor was started)

8. At the end of class, you can quickly tell how much effort the entire class made by looking at the average heart rates and at the total minutes in the target zone. You can also quickly see if students were performing in the extremes—either very low heart rates and little time in the target zone or very high heart rates and several minutes above the target zone. As you can see, heart rate monitors provide instant individual attention and immediate feedback for both you and your students.

9. You can give students wearing a heart rate monitor with a recall/store feature (such as the Polar Accurex II Heart Rate Monitor) throughout class, time credit for average heart rate and minutes in the target zone. If you choose, you can have students or squad leaders record this information in student portfolios daily without downloading to a computer.

Downloading

Using these procedures with a heart rate monitor with a downloading feature, such as the Polar Vantage XL Heart Rate Monitor, helps you provide individual attention and immediate feedback. No one has to wait until the printouts are ready to see the results (see figure 2.2, a-h).

Downloading data from the Polar Vantage XL Heart Rate Monitor provides hardcopy evidence of not only student-by-student heart rate response, but minute-by-minute analysis of each student throughout the physical education class period. This documents a picture of the *structure* of the physical education class time for students,

teachers, parents, administrators, and school board members.

With printouts of heart rates, physical educators who set aside specific segments of class for aerobic development have the means to give all students credit for their personal best efforts. Activity segments of the class time show that some activities provide true gains in cardiovascular benefits, while others do not. This provides clear reasoning for setting aside a specific segment of the physical education class time each day for aerobic development.

Many physical educators have a specific segment of the physical education class time that is used for short lectures or times of specific instructions. Moreover, their time for actual instruction often is restricted because of limited minutes per week and large numbers of students per class. The time constraints for physical educators can be accurately presented for students, teachers, administrators, and school board members alike through the hardcopy printouts that are available for all students who wear the Polar Vantage XL Heart Rate Monitor.

Students are able to personalize their workouts and still be given credit for doing their personal best using the Polar Vantage XL Heart Rate Monitor. Their own printouts from the downloading procedure provide them with the assurance that they will be given credit for doing their personal best. It is important for students to understand why the physical education classes are structured with specifics in mind for certain segments of class. Using their own printouts gives them the personal interest in these discussions. Learning that there is a correct pace that is completely individual for aerobic development is something that only a hardcopy printout from the Polar Vantage XL can deliver. With all students looking at their own printouts during these discussions, it provides the immediate feedback that is a big part of motivation—now and for the future—to establish correct exercise habits within our youth.

Students can download the information themselves starting as early as the fourth grade. However, this will depend on the availability of computers and on the length of physical education classes. Some physical education teachers, like Harold Mercer in Carmel, Indiana, have recruited parent volunteers to download and place the hardcopy printouts in each student's portfolio.

Other physical educators like Harold Spilllman in Overland Park, Kansas, have convinced administrators to provide for a teacher aide for this assistance. Still others, like Rick Shupbach in Grundy Center, Iowa, have the students themselves downloading at the fourth grade level. Pat Roch in Menasha, Wisconsin, downloads all her students' heart rate information beginning with the first grade. Jinks Coleman in Baton Rouge, Louisiana, teaches students in her class how to read the graphs starting in the second grade. Jim Struve and Rhonda Wittmer at Tilford Middle School in Vinton, Iowa, have over 15,000 heart rate printouts from students over the past 15 years. All students there have been using the Polar Vantage XL Heart Rate monitors to record their heart rates not only during class time, but for all mile-run cardiovascular tests given in the fall and again in the spring.

No student has been asked to run the mile cardiovascular test without a Polar Vantage XL Heart Rate Monitor in the past 15 years at Tilford Middle School! Students there are given credit for keeping their heart rates in their target zones throughout the mile run. They also read the graphs and record their pre-exercise heart rates, their times, and their recovery heart rates from their heart rate printouts.

Linda Crawford and Debbie Hunter at Gentry Middle School in Mount Airy, North Carolina, have been using the students' heart rate print-outs for student assignments in which they write a letter to their parents explaining their heart rate graphs. Jan Adair, Director of Physical Education with Fargo, North Dakota schools, says that Karen Roesler, Mary Ann Donnay, and Lois Much are all outstanding physical educators within the Fargo schools who have implemented heart rate monitors throughout their programs using them for assessment, evaluation, and portfolio documentation.

Ball State University in Muncie, Indiana, uses Polar Vantage XL Heart Rate Monitors in over 18 different physical education and wellness courses. Undergraduate physical education majors own their own Polar Vantage XL Heart Rate Monitors and download at the university's physical education computer lab. These students are trained on how to download, analyze printouts, test cardiovascular fitness, individualize conditioning, and keep portfolios.

There are as many ways to use heart rate graph information as their are teachers in this country. It will be exciting to see the results of having the Polar Heart Rate Monitors on the wrists of more and more students across this country and the potential for learning increase in physical education—not only for students, but for teachers, parents, administrators and school board members as well.

Equipment Needs

1. One Polar Vantage XL Heart Rate Monitor for each student
2. One Polar Interface System and computer for each student

If you do not have enough monitors for each student, divide the class into two groups and rotate which group is using the monitors every other physical education day. Two may share one computer using the Polar Interface System, but you must allow more class time for downloading. The research shows that students learn more about computer use when they work in pairs, rather than alone. Also, a more adept student can help a less adept student, actually saving both the teacher's time and class time. Each student will need one to two minutes to download his or her heart rate information from the heart rate monitor and to save the information for printing out later for inclusion in individual portfolios. This will also be the procedure for the assessment of the cardiovascular test, using the mile run or the nine-minute run.

Procedures

1. Upon receiving a heart rate monitor, have each student warm up and then start the monitor in the recording mode and begin the exercise portion of class. Once the students have received their heart rate monitors and turned them on, you can teach class without interruption.
2. At the end of class, signal all students to continue to cool down until their heart rates have dropped to the safe cool-down heart rate zone (see chart for each age group). After cooling down, have students once again line up in squads, waiting for your

instructions. The warm-up and cool-down times will not be calculated in the target heart rate zone because they will fall below this target zone.

3. You may find it helpful to post the following instructions on the wall behind each computer so that students may read them as they wait for a turn to download.

Instructions for Students

After you have loaded the software and prepared the computer for downloading, provide these instructions for students to download.

1. Push the set/start/stop button once.
2. Push the select button once.
3. Push the set/start/stop button once. At this point the Polar Vantage XL Heart Rate Monitor should read "Comp."
4. Push the store/recall (red button) once. At this point, the heart rate monitor should read 1 to 8, depending on the file number.
5. Go to the computer and set your Polar Vantage XL Heart Rate Monitor on the Polar Interface (small black box) and press the store/recall button once. The computer should say that the information is being received, and the heart rate monitor should show the "Comp" blinking.
6. Once this information is received by the computer, the heart rate monitor will beep.
7. You may then see a graph of the information by going to "Curve" under the "View" pull-down menu.
8. Students should then save the file using initials and class number. (Of course, you should train these students ahead of time on how to save files.)

Heart Rate Portfolios

Classroom teachers in various subject areas have had their students create portfolios in which to place examples of their best class work. In their physical education portfolios, students may appropriately be asked to include written examples of their fitness goals and plans, daily nutritional intakes, exercise notes, and personal observations of effort. The heart rate printouts from the Polar

Vantage XL are the only hardcopy data giving actual personal documentation of participation during class time. The printouts from the mile run or other cardiovascular tests may later become invaluable information, and they should be kept for each student in a portfolio throughout their school years. The information from actual class time, using heart rate response and the time line, produce objective authentic assessments that credit each student for effort that might otherwise only be observed subjectively.

Students will use the Polar Vantage XL printouts to record the percentage of time they spend in the target zone during each class period. They should also specify what activities produced the highest percentage of class time in the target zone. Students will compare heart rate printouts for the mile run or nine-minute run in the fall and spring to see if improvement in time or yardage occurred and to look for consistent heart rates on both tests to ensure they expend consistent effort or intensity. They will also use their pre-exercise heart rates from the fall and spring tests to figure the various heart rate zones and determine their individual target zones. Students can include homework assignments in their portfolios when printouts have been received and then can reflect on these efforts.

After the information has been downloaded, you may evaluate portfolios and compare heart rates and different activities by comparing the printouts (see figure 2.2, *a-h*).

You can use the heart rate information to answer many questions, such as the following:

1. In each of the physical education classes, did the student follow the recommended format of gradual warm-up, sustained heart rate in the target zone, and cool-down?
2. Following the warm-up, which activity sustained the heart rate in the target zone the longest?
3. Which activities were not effective in sustaining the heart rate in the target zone? Activities often require cardiovascular fitness, but do not develop it.

You can also compare the relative efforts of students based on heart rate information. The graphs in figure 2.3 show multiple file summaries for two different students performing the same activities.

Questions for Thought

1. What are three observations that you can draw from these comparisons?
2. Since no two students are alike, does the chart surprise you?

3. Explain how students could adjust their exercising, according to the science of heart rate information.
4. How could you adjust what you are doing to encourage more consistent benefits for every student in every lesson?

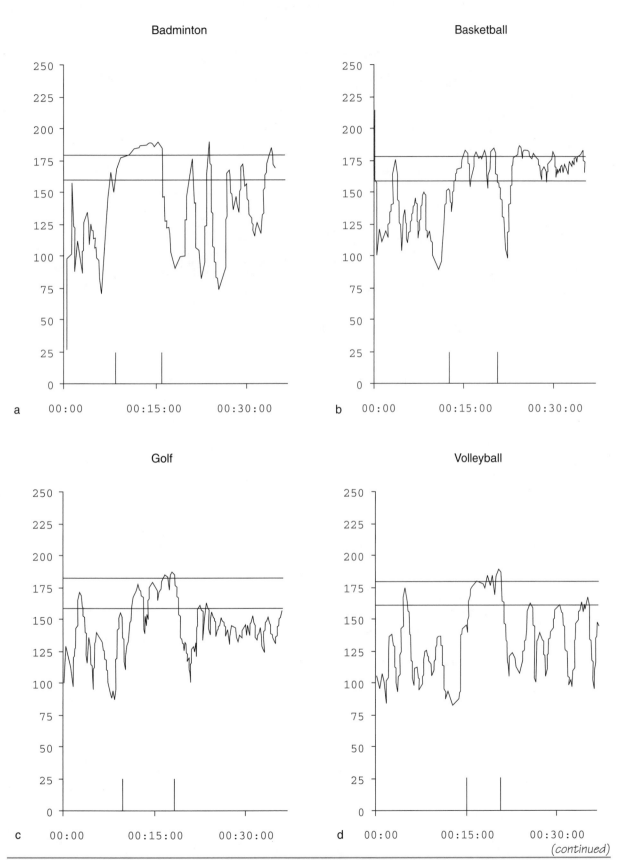

Figure 2.2 During the aerobic segment of class, marked by the solid vertical lines on the bottom of the graph, the heart rate monitor records the activity portion of the class.

(continued)

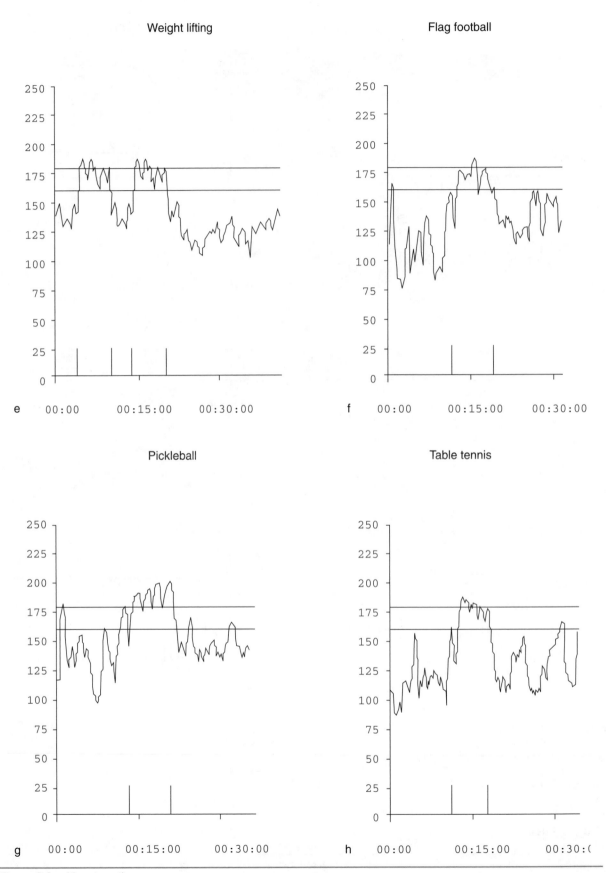

Figure 2.2 *(Continued).*

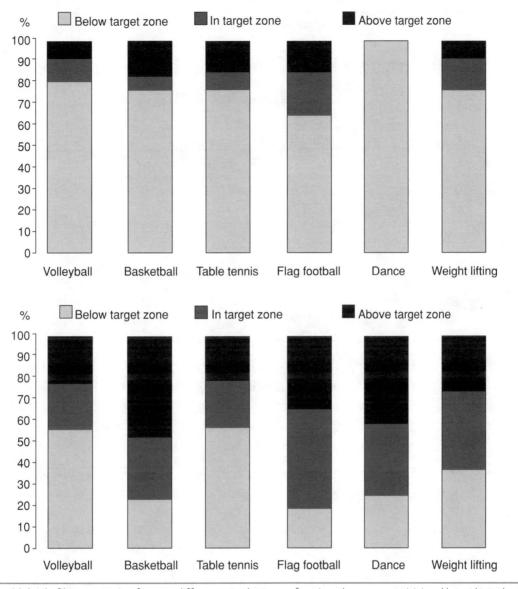

Figure 2.3 Multiple file summaries for two different students performing the same activities. Note that the lower graphs show that the student received greater cardiovascular benefit than the student in the upper graphs.

Macintosh Helpful Hints to Showcase Polar Graphs and Printouts

You can cut and paste as many as three Polar graphs onto one page if you use the "picture-taking" capabilities of the Macintosh.

1. Simply take a picture by opening the Polar heart rate file of any student (double-click on the file name).

2. Arrow over to "View."

3. Open each of the graphs you wish to paste onto a word processor file.

4. As you open each graph, simply press the apple key, the shift key, and the number 3 key at the same time, and you will hear a click. This indicates that a picture has been taken of that screen. It will be listed as "Picture 1" on the hard drive of your computer.

5. You may rename that picture by clicking on "Picture 1" and renaming it as the file it represents, such as "Kirkpatrick, Beth—VB," telling you that it was Beth Kirkpatrick's volleyball physical education class that the heart rate data reflects.

6. When you have taken a picture of the two or three graphs that you want for that student, one by one, copy and paste these picture to the document that you want. You do not need to copy the entire screen. You may wish to copy only a portion of the screen. By holding down the button that is the clicker, you can select the section of the screen you want to copy (see figure 2.4, a and b). Notice that we have copied and pasted two separate graphs to a single page. We can move this same information to other documents or even print it.

```
Time          Heart rate values
00:00:00   75 111 124 103  92  73  72  77  77  93  79  75
00:03:00   75  80  74  87  79  81  80  81  73  85  87  84
00:06:00   82  82  81  79  89  87  92  98  95  96 106 100
00:09:00  108 127 134 125 102  90  91  85  85  85  86  87
00:12:00  101  87  88 116 109  99  90  84  97 101 102  90
00:15:00   84  87 102  92  92  86  87  93  98  95 136 133
00:18:00  143 143 160 175 170 146 146 133 156 155 136 125
00:21:00  117 128 127 158 155 152 139 126 139 144 130 118
00:24:00  108 124 114 108 111 111 111 166 184 187 190 192
00:27:00  190 192 192 197 194 198 195 194 194 193 195 197
00:30:00  196 196 195 196 197 197 197 196 198 196 195 196
00:33:00  195 193 190 191 189 179 170 164 158 136 129 105
00:36:00  109  97 102 108  99 100  98  98 106  96  88  84
00:39:00   94 104 110 137 146 143 142 141 134 126 156 145
00:42:00  139 126 104 117 119 119 119 124 114 114 123 129
00:45:00  142 130 131 145 157 171 175 169 164 163 161 153
```

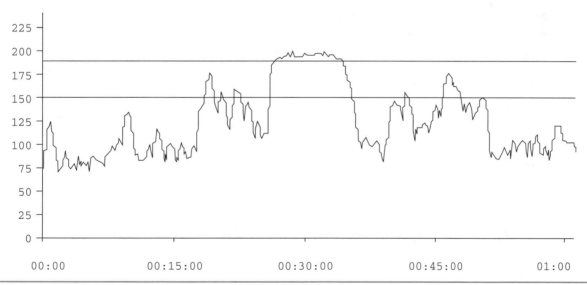

Figure 2.4a   The student's heart rate listing and the student's graph of the heart rate are able to be printed on one sheet of paper so you may write a note on the paper as well as give, explain, or summarize the results.

Time	Heart rate values											
00:00:00	75	111	124	103	92	73	72	77	77	93	79	75
00:03:00	75	80	74	87	79	81	80	81	73	85	87	84
00:06:00	82	82	81	79	89	87	92	98	95	96	106	100
00:09:00	108	127	134	125	102	90	91	85	85	85	86	87
00:12:00	101	87	88	116	109	99	90	84	97	101	102	90
00:15:00	84	87	102	92	92	86	87	93	98	95	136	133
00:18:00	143	143	160	175	170	146	146	133	156	155	136	125
00:21:00	117	128	127	158	155	152	139	126	139	144	130	118
00:24:00	108	124	114	108	111	111	111	166	184	187	190	192
00:27:00	190	192	192	197	194	198	195	194	194	193	195	197
00:30:00	196	196	195	196	197	197	197	196	198	196	195	196
00:33:00	195	193	190	191	189	179	170	164	158	136	129	105
00:36:00	109	97	102	108	99	100	98	98	106	96	88	84
00:39:00	94	104	110	137	146	143	142	141	134	126	156	145
00:42:00	139	126	104	117	119	119	119	124	114	114	123	129
00:45:00	142	130	131	145	157	171	175	169	164	163	161	153

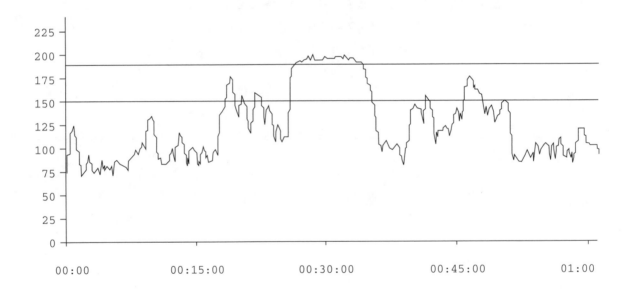

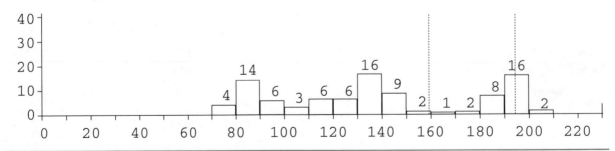

Figure 2.4b Using Macintosh computers, you may move the graphs to other documents, as well as copy and paste, once you take "pictures" of the graphs.

CHAPTER

3

Getting Started With Heart Rate Monitors

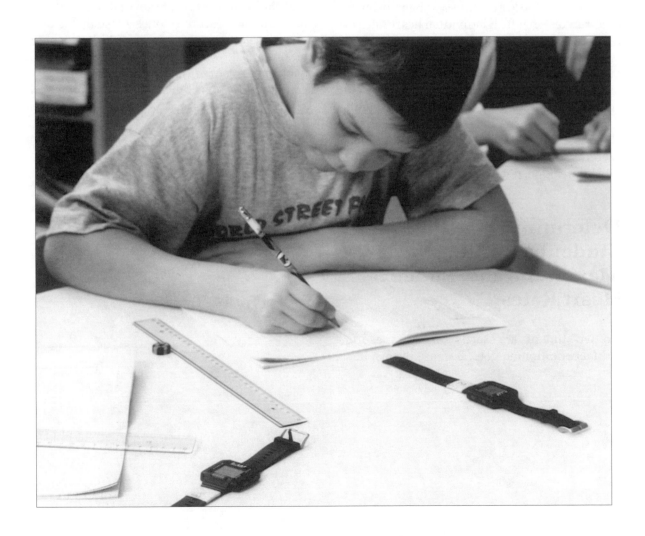

Asking students to do the best they can has always been one of the basic goals of physical education. Yet, we've never had an objective way to document student by student the success or failure of this goal, day to day. Even more importantly, asking students to make their best efforts but not being able to provide the immediate and continuous feedback has made authentic assessment difficult, if not impossible.

Throughout this chapter, you and your students will begin to explore the ramifications of understanding heart rate information. The immediate feedback will provide you with the potential for giving clear and safe instructions to each student, based on individual heart rate responses to lessons. In the very first lesson, your students will begin to see that resting heart rates are individual and vary from day to day, student to student. After using heart rate monitors for several days in physical education, your students will be excited about the lesson on assessment, using the mile-run test in which individual heart rates determine correct intensity (mile-run pacing)—not an instructor's subjective interpretation of how fast each student should run without knowledge of anyone's heart rate. All students will find a new era has emerged in physical education in which using a heart rate monitor ensures that accountability and instruction rely on the applications of exercise science to each individual, using heart rate knowledge, not guesswork.

Determining Each Student's Resting, Maximum, and Target Heart Rates

No two students are exactly alike as far as individual conditioning goes. Because of this, heart rates among students participating in the same activity may vary throughout the activity or at different stages of the activity. Heart rate monitors help you individualize each student's conditioning regimen. To determine the correct range for each student's heart rate during exercise, figure the target heart rate zone for each individual. The formula includes knowing the maximum and resting heart rates and age of each individual. Remember, you can calculate your resting heart rate by checking your pulse as soon as you wake up in the morning, before you lift your head from the pillow. Determine your maximum heart rate by subtracting your age from 220. Then you can figure the target heart rate zone using the Karvonen formula (see explanation in chapter 5, lesson 7) or a number of other heart rate formulas (see the example in chapter 2). Since several different heart rate zones and several different ways to determine those zones exist, it is important that you incorporate several different ways to figure the heart rate zones. Once that is determined, heart rate monitors provide the documentation and the continuous individualized feedback that ensures that students will be given credit and responsibility for conditioning at the correct levels.

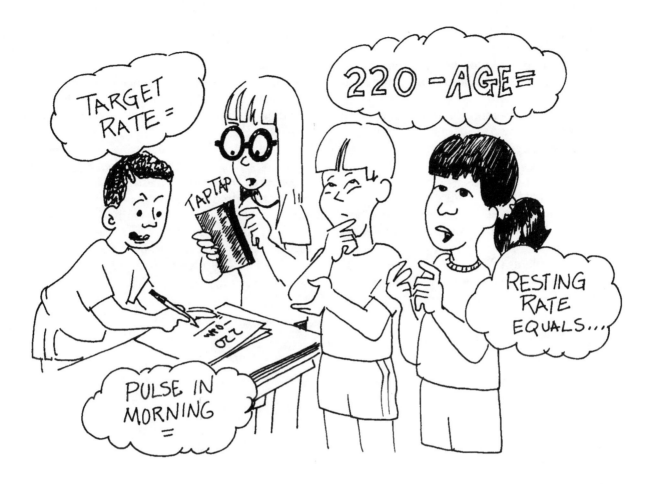

Lesson 1

Science and Resting Heart Rate

Students must calculate and know their resting heart rates to effectively use heart rate monitors for physical fitness.

Goals:

- To learn how to take an accurate resting heart rate.
- To learn that resting heart rates do vary from day to day and to understand the need to sometimes change an individual conditioning program accordingly because of how resting heart rate affects the target heart rate zone.

Key Concepts:

Resting heart rates can vary from day to day. Overtraining, stress, drugs, sickness, and lack of a consistent conditioning program are some of the factors that can affect changes day to day in resting heart rates.

Materials:

- One heart rate monitor for each student
- Large area in which all students are able to lie down
- One worksheet 3.1 for each student

Activity:

1. Have students put on heart rate monitors and find a place to lie down on the gym floor or bleachers.
2. Have students monitor their heart rates while lying down for 10 minutes to see how low they can get them. Every minute, have students make their heart rate monitors store their heart rates.
3. At the end of the 10 minutes, have students recall their 10 heart rates from their monitors and record the 6 lowest heart rates on worksheet 3.1.
4. Have students take their heart rates manually for six consecutive days at home, following the directions on worksheet 3.1.

Teaching Tips:

The worksheet may be more appropriate for upper elementary or middle school students. High school students may be more receptive to creating their own resting heart rate reports or heart rate journals.

Inhalers may elevate heart rates, so discuss this with your students and how adjustments in exercise must be made for asthma as well as for other individual needs. Point out that heart rates can be affected without an individual's knowledge. Heart rate monitors provide continuous feedback, allowing each individual the opportunity to adjust to exercise safely and correctly every day.

Notes

Instructions:

1. After taking your resting heart rate every minute for 10 consecutive minutes at school, record the six lowest heart rates across the "HR school" row in table 3.1 below. Find the average of the heart rates by adding the numbers together and dividing by six.

2. Make sure you are healthy and are having a "normal" week (meaning no extremely stressful situations). Then do the following for the next six days at home: After the alarm wakes you in the morning, wait one to two minutes and take your pulse for 60 seconds. (Do not take it for 15 seconds and multiply by four. If you are off one heart beat then your 60-second score will be 4 beats off!) Do this for six mornings and record your scores in table 3.1 across the "HR home" row. To find your average heart rate, total the six days' records of resting heart rate and divide by six.

TABLE 3.1   Heart Rate Normal Variability Test

	1	2	3	4	5	6	Average
Date							
HR school							
HR home							

Use the information you have collected to answer the following questions:

1. On what day did you record the lowest resting heart rate?

2. What is an excellent resting heart rate?

3. Was your resting heart rate the same every day?

4. What are some reasons why resting heart rate may be higher some days than other days?

5. What are some reasons why some people have higher resting heart rates and other people have lower resting heart rates?

6. Compare the resting heart rates of five other students in your class. What is the average resting heart rate of the five students?

   What is the average heart rate?

   What was the lowest?

   What was the highest?

(continued)

7. Graph your resting heart rate for six days in a row. What was the average resting heart rate for these six days?

   What was the lowest?

   What was the highest?

8. Asthma is a common affliction in America. What does the use of an inhaler *do* to the resting heart rate?

   Why is knowledge of heart rate for those who have asthma and who exercise important?

9. Does pop or coffee affect your heart rate and your sleep?
10. Do your nerves affect heart rate?
11. How does regular aerobic exercise affect the resting heart rate? Why?

12. Do muscular people automatically have lower resting heart rates than less muscular people?
13. Is it better to have a lower or higher resting heart rate? Why?

14. What time of day is really the most accurate for finding your resting heart rate?

Lesson 2

Finding Your Maximum Heart Rate and Target Heart Rate Zone

Effective physical fitness lessons using heart rate monitors require students to know what their maximum heart rates should be so they can then calculate their target heart rate zones.

Goals:

- To learn how to calculate maximum heart rate and target heart rate.
- To understand that age is a variable in the formula for finding target heart rate zones and that this is why their parents' target heart rate zones are very different from their own.
- To understand that the Karvonen formula adds resting heart rate as a variable that defines a more individualized zone.
- To allow the student to be personally accountable for their cardiovascular efforts by staying within their target zone.

Key Concepts:

Age is a main factor in figuring maximum heart rates, target heart rate zones, and resting heart rates. Each day's workout is determined by heart rate response—that is why heart rate knowledge during a workout is important. It gives an individual the feedback to either speed up or slow down accordingly.

Materials:

- One heart rate monitor for each student
- Calculators (optional)
- One worksheet 3.2 for each student

Activity:

1. Have the students subtract their age from 220. This is the estimated maximum heart rate. (Chapter 5, lesson 7 shows how to figure the maximum heart rate using the Karvonen formula, which also figures in resting heart rate and is slightly more accurate.)

2. Have each student multiply the maximum heart rate by .70 to get an approximate target heart rate. This is the lower limit of the target zone. Then have each student multiply the first number by .85 to calculate the higher heart rate limit of the target zone.

The following shows the correct calculations for a 14-year-old female or male:

$$220 - 14 \ = 206$$
$$206 \times .70 = 144.20$$
$$206 \times .85 = 175.10$$

Thus, the estimated target heart rate zone for a 14-year-old is 144 to 175 beats per minute.

3. Have students fill out worksheet 3.2. If you are using the Karvonen formula, multiply by .60 and .80 to find the range for target heart rate.

Teaching Tips:

- Ask students if their parents exercise and know what their heart rates should be before, during, and after exercise.
- Ask students if they think it is important for adults to know their proper heart rate zones for exercise.
- Ask students to plan an open house during which all parents and grandparents could use heart rate monitors and learn their heart rate responses before, during, and after exercise.
- Ask students to take the worksheet home and have an adult fill it out.
- You could use worksheet 3.2 in parts: part I for the first part of the school year and part II for later in the year or for extra credit after the students have been using heart rate monitors for awhile.
- Depending on the ages and abilities of the students, you may wish to allow them to use calculators to figure their target zones.

Figuring Maximum Heart Rate and Target Heart Rate Zones

Reminders:

Maximum heart rate = 220 − (age of subject)

Target heart rate zone = maximum heart rate $\times$ .70

maximum heart rate $\times$ .85

Example:

Marcus is 10 years old.

To find his maximum heart rate the equation looks like this:

220 − 10 = 210

His maximum heart rate is 210 beats per minute.

To find his target heart rate zone the equations look like this:

210 (.70) = 147 beats per minute

210 (.85) = 178.5 beats per minute

Marcus's target heart rate zone is between 147 and 178.50 beats per minute. Marcus should keep his heart rate between 147 and 178.50 beats per minute during physical activity.

Part I

1. Figure the target heart rate zone for one of your teachers.

2. Figure the target heart rate zone for one of your parents.

3. Figure the target heart rate zone for the oldest person you know.

4. List three types of activities in which you have participated in physical education class that have raised your heart rate into your target zone according to your heart rate portfolio.

(continued)

Part II

1. List three types of activities in which you have participated in physical education class that have not raised your heart rate into your target heart rate zone.

2. What is one type of activity outside school that would raise your heart rate into your target heart rate zone?

3. What is the one factor that makes the target heart rate zone different for you, one of your parents, and one of your grandparents?

4. Ask five different people to give you their target heart rate zones. If they do not know, record this and figure it out for them. Were you surprised that they did not know how to figure their target heart rate zones?

   What were their reactions to your question?

   Were they happy to know their target heart rate zones after you figured it for them?

   How should they use this information?

5. Look at one of your heart rate printouts and estimate how many minutes you were in your target heart rate zone. Attach that printout to this worksheet.

6. Using a heart rate monitor, record the minutes you were in the target heart rate zone for each physical education class. Find the total minutes you spent in the target heart rate zone for one month. What was the average total of minutes you were in the target heart rate zone during each physical education class? (Divide the number of total minutes for the month by the number of classes you attended.)

Mile-Run Test: Evaluating Fitness Gains

The mile-run test (and the nine-minute test, which similarly allows for documenting consistent effort through heart rate monitoring) often is designed to be performed in the fall and again in the spring. Typically students whose time decreases by the spring are determined to have improved their cardiovascular fitness since the fall. Until recently, however, student's heart rates have not been taken before, during, or after the mile-run test. Without knowing heart rates, how can this test be accurate, safe, or provide children with the awareness that heart rate is an important indicator of correct intensity throughout the test?

Many students still graduate from high school never having had the immediate feedback of their heart rates during exercise or testing even though weather conditions may vary, such as high heat and humidity, and health conditions may vary, based on the individual. It is no wonder that few adults have used heart rate to determine intensity of exercise! During their kindergarten through 12th grade education, they were probably never encouraged to keep track of their heart rates during exercise or, even worse, during cardiovascular testing in physical education.

With this in mind, we have introduced a mile-run test that utilizes the Polar Vantage XL Heart Rate Monitor. This heart rate monitor provides immediate feedback throughout testing as well as a printout with complete statistical analysis for every student each time she wears the heart rate monitor. Figure 3.1 shows a printout of the fall and spring mile-run test for one student. Resting heart rate, recovery heart rate, and a consistent level of intensity according to the heart rate is verified for both fall and spring tests. The only variables are the time and maturation; thus the cardiovascular improvement is clearly visible and measurable.

To perform this test accurately, you must hold each student accountable for sustaining her heart rate within the upper limits of the target heart rate zone. If the student does not sustain her heart rate in that zone throughout the mile run, require her to run the mile again the next class and each class thereafter until her heart rate is sustained in the upper limits of the zone throughout the test. The emphasis on staying in the target zone, rather than on maximum effort, eliminates the variability of results due to differences in students' efforts. Use heart rate monitors in this structured and proven way to document consistency and individualization of effort requirements for the mile-run or nine-minute cardiovascular test. The student with a higher percent body fat will now have the technology to provide the safe feedback that very likely will give that person "permission" to walk. Don't ask students to run the mile without heart rate knowledge.

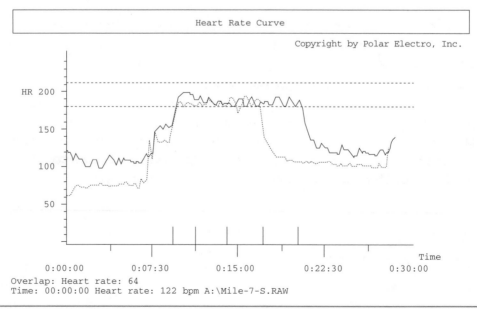

Figure 3.1   Resting heart rate decreased, mile time decreased, and recovery was faster in spring (dotted presentation showing marked improvements with constant effort).

Lesson 3

Mile-Run Test

Using heart rate monitors, you can safely and accurately administer the mile-run or nine-minute run cardiovascular tests in the fall and again in the spring.

Goals:

- To hold the heart rate in the upper limits of the target zone throughout the test in both the fall and spring test.
- To test safely throughout the school physical education experience, teaching that heart rate is the most important factor in testing for cardiovascular conditioning.

Key Concepts:

Students need to understand that sustaining the correct heart rate throughout the run is the most important objective of this test. Encourage them to run along the inside of the track throughout the test in both the fall and the spring. Some students will try to run several steps to the outside of the inner circle, actually running much farther than a mile; this can affect results if they run on the inside of the track during one test but on the outside during the other test. Stagger-start students to avoid competition. Nobody wants to be the last to finish. Remember, the times are being individually recorded by each heart rate monitor, so you don't need to start all students together. Explain that for the test to be accurate, the student must hold heart rate in the same target zone in both the fall test and the spring test. To show a true gain in cardiovascular fitness, the time in the spring mile must have dropped.

Materials:

- One heart rate monitor for each student
- Stopwatch
- Clipboard with time chart
- Pencil

Activity:

1. As each student receives a heart rate monitor, have him immediately find a space to lie down and relax for at least five minutes. Some students will be resting longer than others but all should remain in the resting position for at least five minutes.
2. While the students are in the gym resting, provide them with information such as telling them to make sure they run close to the inside of the track, maintain the heart rate in the target zone, try to keep a constant pace that only heart rate can determine, and run four laps, then continue to walk for a set distance for the cool-down.
3. Have students run the mile run, keeping within their target heart rate zones. Instruct anyone running above her target heart rate (signaled by the monitor beeping) to walk until her heart rate reaches the lower limit of the target zone, then resume running.
4. The monitor times and records each student's mile time. Have students walk to cool down until their heart rates stop decreasing or their heart rate has dropped 40 beats.
5. After resting for five minutes after the cool-down, have students check their heart rate monitors, then return them to you.
6. In the spring, repeat the process. By overlapping with computer graphics the fall mile with the spring mile, you can measure and compare cardiovascular fitness according to heart rate. Three indicators to look at are resting heart rate, recovery heart rate, and the mile time that is established according to heart rate (effort). Each of these indicators improves (decreases) as an individual becomes more cardiovascularly fit.
7. Use worksheets 3.3 and 3.4 to teach students how to read their heart rate printouts from the tests.

Teaching Tips:

Running groups: Using the results from the mile-run or nine-minute test, determine running groups. For example, if three students ran nine-minute miles (within 15 seconds) and held their heart rates in the target zone, and their pre-exercise heart rates were within 10 beats of each other, these students are of similar fitness and ability, and you should group them together. Then, if your equipment ratio of heart rate monitors to students is not one to one, you may put one heart rate monitor on one of the partners in each running group and use this to determine correct pacing for all students in the group. If one or more of the students seems to be having trouble with that pace, we advise placing heart rate monitors on those students as well to determine if their conditioning has changed over the course of several weeks. Yet, monitoring concerns such as stress, drug use, and overtraining is best-served by equipping each student with a heart rate monitor.

Partner system: Each partner has a transmitter belt on and one partner wears the heart rate monitor for the first half of the class and the other for the second half. Each set of partners sets a goal for number of minutes of their combined efforts for the heart rate to be in the target zone. Be sure to have one partner press the store/recall button when the second partner's turn to use the heart monitor begins. Calculate the total minutes that the team was in the target zone and calculate each partner's total minutes in the target zone. Do not give credit for being too high or too low (outside the target zone). Do this activity for several days. Then ask your students the following questions:

- Did each student contribute equally to the team heart rate totals?
- How do you feel when you are contributing the most?
- How do you feel when you do not contribute the same as the other partner?
- Whose responsibility is it to earn a fair share of the credit?
- Why do you think that in team activities some people often do not carry their fair share of the load?
- How can you help change this?

Notes

Learning to Read Graphs From the Nine-Minute Test

1. Circle the graph below that shows the heart rate too low.
2. Draw a "♡" on the graphs that show the tests with heart rates held steadily in the target zone.
3. Between the two graphs with the "♡," which graph shows the lowest recovery heart rate?
4. Draw an "X" through the graph that shows the test done with the heart rate not held steady.
5. If the heart rate had been too low in the fall test and at the right level for the spring test, would the results be a true test of improvement?

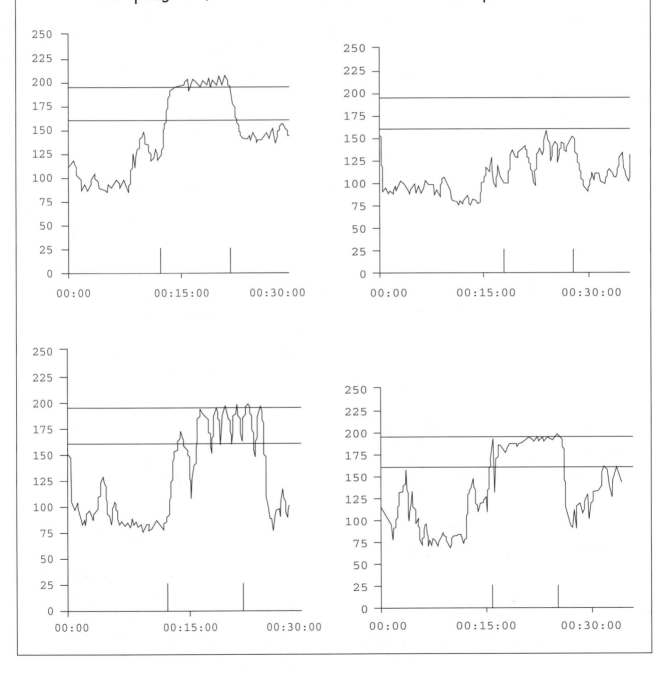

Understanding Heart Rate Graphs From the Mile-Run Test

If the heart rate is held consistently within the target zone in the fall and in the spring test, then the improvement in time is truly an indicator for cardiovascular improvement.

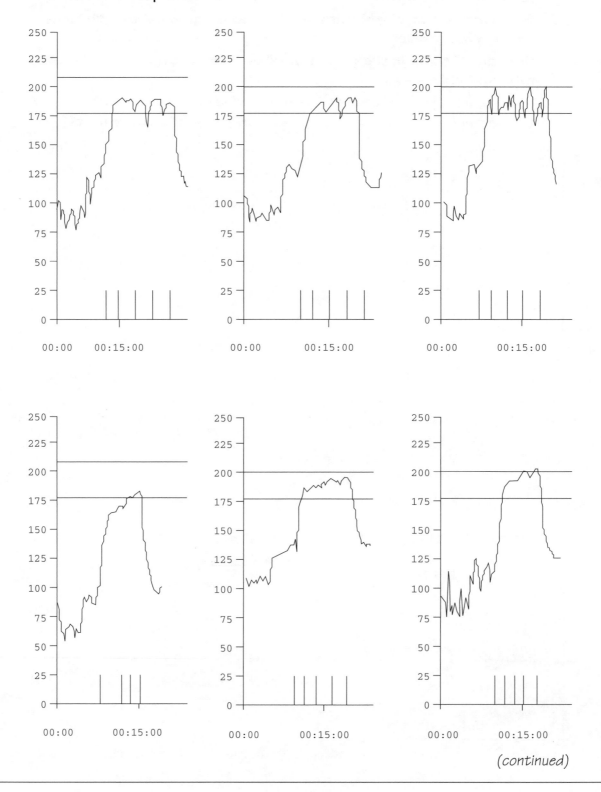

(continued)

Worksheet 3.4

1. Draw a "♡" on the graph that shows the highest resting heart rate.

2. Draw a square on the graph that shows the most irregular heart rate during the mile-run test.

3. Place an "X" on the graph that shows the student who did not run the four laps required for the test.

4. Draw a triangle on the graph that shows a very high heart rate throughout the mile.

5. Circle the graphs that show the mile-run test has been completed correctly.

Class Heart Rates: Accountability Using Heart Rate Monitors

We have never had a scientific tool that documented what effort has been given by each student for each lesson. If grades are to be given based in some part on effort, then we should have some objective measurement of effort. Using heart rate monitors, you can evaluate the lessons you teach in terms of effort and activity, based on the percentage of time students were in the target zones. If many students were at low levels, you should look at the lesson or other factors to see where you can improve consistency and motivation. If you plan to give students credit for their efforts, the heart rate information can document this, often providing clear proof that students are or are not doing their best as individuals. Either way, you and your students will have a basic understanding that information is being gathered lesson by lesson, student by student, providing a means of accountability for both students and teachers.

Questions for Thought

1. List the average heart rate of students in each class or activity using heart rate monitors.
2. Encourage each physical education teacher in your school to do the same.
3. Which activity produced the highest average heart rate?
4. Which activity produced the lowest average heart rate?
5. Was there a class that consistently averaged higher heart rates? If so, what could be some of the reasons? What was the percentage of time spent in the target zone?
6. Compare classes with same and different teachers doing the same activity. Did some of the teachers' physical education classes have student heart rate averages consistently higher than other classes of theirs or other teachers? Did the time of day of class affect the average heart rates? Why or why not?

7. Does the format of the class help determine higher or lower class average heart rates?
8. Is too much time spent on lecturing or too little? Evaluate the format according to the heart rate monitor printouts using the Polar Vantage XL Heart Rate Monitor and determine if you can document consistent format in teaching style, such as 5 minutes spent on warm-up exercises, 10 minutes spent on aerobic development, 20 minutes spent on activity, 3 minutes spent on closure activity, cool-down, and so on.
9. If the information from the heart rate monitors shows that one class is consistently lower in average heart rates than others or one school's average heart rates are much lower, some problems could be not having enough equipment, having class sizes too large for area provided, poorly designed lessons that create lines in which students stand around, inefficient structure of transitions or getting started, too many team members on teams, activities not aerobically designed, or students disinterested because of competitive factors, size differentiation, coed or lack of coed classes, athletic versus nonathletic members in class makeup causing friction or domination of one group, intimidation, frustration in drills, and the like.

Physical educators have often been unfairly represented by those who fail to provide quality programs. Students also have often been unfairly evaluated subjectively for effort throughout each activity and for "perceived" intensity during the cardiovascular tests traditionally given in the fall and spring. Heart rate monitors may be the one invention that paints a true picture of each person's efforts throughout physical education classes. Moreover, the heart rate monitors may bring physical educators the accountability that many other areas of education already have received. Everyone can receive credit, and you and your students can both document accountability—a boon in this age of authentic assessment!

Beginner Lesson Plans

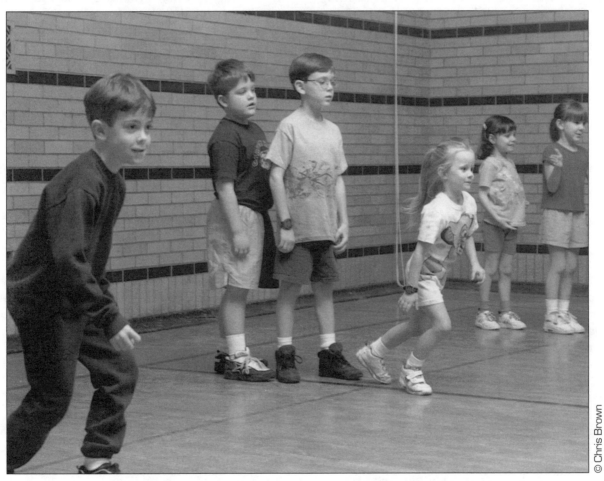

© Chris Brown

All students delight in the use of technology, especially when it pertains to their own bodies. By using the heart rate monitors at the elementary level, students begin at a young age to see that heart rates provide the tool for exercising at the right level each day. Many times, elementary physical education teachers expect students to exercise and move without regard to heart rate. It is especially important to reassure children using technology that each student will receive credit for doing the best they can. This removes the fear of failure, reassuring all students that they can succeed in terms of effort.

Lesson 1
Seasons of the Heart

Using a heart rate monitor, this careful recording of the heart rate during the resting, warm-up, exercise, and cool-down stages can teach safe training practices.

Goals:

- To see that exercising correctly means including the four parts of exercise: resting, warm-up, exercise, and cool-down.
- To associate the seasons of nature with the seasons of the heart and the natural workout process, using these steps every time you exercise.

Key Concepts:

All workouts should be preceded by a warm-up that gradually increases the heart rate through a series of stretching and large muscle movements. Once the muscles have been properly warmed through increased blood flow and heart rate, the body is ready to experience the exercise heart rate, taking the heart into a sustained target heart rate zone appropriate for the age and condition of the individual. Every workout should include careful monitoring of the resting heart rate, the warm-up heart rate, the exercise heart rate, and the recovery heart rate. Tell students "As the seasons follow the same progression each year, remember the importance of using a warm-up and cool-down period each time you exercise—like nature."

Materials:

- Heart rate monitors with downloading capabilities (such as the Polar Vantage XL Heart Rate Monitor) for each student
- Computer access

Activity:

1. Attach the heart rate monitor and have the students warm up for 10 minutes or until the heart rate reaches 135 beats per minute.
2. Complete the exercise section of the class.
3. Once the exercise period is finished, allow for a gradual slowing down of the heart rate by engaging in continuous movement such as walking for several minutes.
4. Have each student download her heart rate information. You will need to do this for younger students.

Teaching Tips:

Create a bulletin board about the seasons of the year. Tie the students' heart rate monitor printouts in with the season's theme.

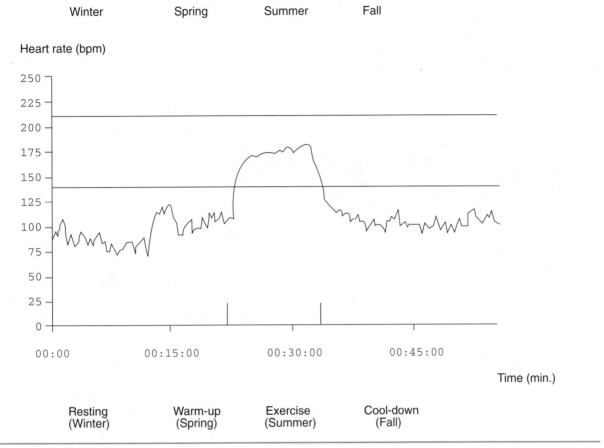

Figure 4.1 *Seasons of the heart.*

_____ Notes _____

Lesson 2
Heart Rate Bingo

This activity is appropriate for students of all ages. The Polar Accurex II Heart Rate Monitors supply an individual's average heart rate throughout class by pushing a button. Each day, the potential for a different number is quite high. The heart rate bingo card provides students with the motivation to check their average heart rates each day they play the game. This helps you progressively place more responsibility for staying interested in their own heart rates on the students. While playing heart rate bingo, students become increasingly interested in taking their heart rates as they fill in their bingo cards. As their excitement builds, they begin to take more responsibility for tracking their heart rates.

Goals:

- To know and check on their average heart rates throughout the school year for every physical education day.
- To recognize that different activities elicit different heart rates throughout class.
- To understand that heart rates indicate personal effort and are therefore their responsibility to maintain; the Polar Accurex II Heart Rate Monitors, which provide continuous readings throughout class, will help them in this regard.

Key Concepts:

Using average heart rates, students can see that heart rates are individual and that they can use heart rate information both for fun and for knowing if exercise is appropriate for their age and condition.

Materials:

- Bingo cards (see sample on page 43) and pens or pencils for each student

- One heart rate monitor (such as Polar Accurex II HRM) for each student

Activity:

1. Give every student one heart rate bingo card every nine weeks.
2. Each day, have each student wear the heart rate monitor during physical education class. At the end of physical education class, have each student find the average heart rate, and if it matches any one of the numbers on the card, he can cross out that number.
3. Tell students that when they have one row that is crossed out either vertically, horizontally, or diagonally they can bring the card to you to check. If a student's numbers match the numbers that you have recorded each day, give the student heart rate bingo credits that she can use or accumulate for various awards.
4. If any student achieves a "black out" in which all squares are marked, give that student special recognition in the form of a special award.

Teaching Tips:

- Challenge the students to team with another student to challenge other partner teams either in their own class or other classes.
- Teachers should devise multiple bingo cards so that the same configuration of numbers is not used over and over. When you make your own card, be sure all numbers are within the safe target heart rate zones for your students.

	H	E	A	L	T	H	Y
H	145	135	147	134	150	144	130
E	133	125	157	140	141	159	160
A	160	151	131	Know your heart rate!	130	156	171
R	166	145	161	155	142	143	175
T	152	164	153	143	162	137	169
S	148	154	168	170	128	161	164

— *Notes* —

Lesson 3

Listen for the Beat of Your Heart

This lesson focuses on listening skills, following teacher's instructions, basic locomotor movements, and using heart rate monitors safely for individualized cardiovascular conditioning.

Goals:

- To move to the beat of their own hearts.
- To see that others' heart rates are not the same as theirs, understanding both that this is why they must use their own hearts and that learning is an individual experience.
- To see the correlation between heart rate and the concept of exercise intensity.

Key Concepts:

Students will move according to their heart rates because they can see and hear their heart rate by using individual heart rate monitors.

Materials:

- One heart rate monitor for each student

Activity:

1. Program the heart rate target zone into each monitor before class to prevent loss of class time. (For this activity the general zone should fall between 150 to 195 beats per minute for elementary students and 140 to 165 for high school students.)
2. Assign each student a heart rate monitor.
3. Instruct students to listen to the beat of their own hearts via the heart rate monitors.
4. Tell students not to leave the gym, or if outside, clearly mark and describe the areas that are safe.
5. When you give the signal, indicate that students are free to begin moving for 10 min-

utes in any direction they want by skipping, galloping, running, or hopping—taking their heart rates to the upper number of their target zone until it beeps.
6. Each time they hear their heart monitor beeping, insist that they change direction and walk until the heart monitor begins beeping again.
7. Each time a student's monitor beeps after walking, she must again change direction and move again, either skipping, galloping, running, or hopping, until her heart monitor begins beeping again, signaling her to walk again, and so on.
8. Ask the students the following questions:
   - Could you copy someone else, switching directions when they did?
   - Why not?
   - When did your heart rate speed up?
   - When did it slow down?
   - Did anyone have exactly the same movements at the same time?
   - Do you think your heart rate is important to know?
   - Whose heart rate should you listen to, yours or your friend's?

Teaching Tips:

Teach students the vocabulary of fast and slow using heart rate monitors which provide instant and continuous visual and auditory feedback. You can also have the students clap to the beat of their hearts or to alternate raising their right and left hands in time to the beeping of their heart rate monitors during this exercise. Point out that some students' heart rates (claps, rising arms) are going faster than others and some students' heart rates are going slower than others. Be sure to point out the recovery heart rate and how it relates to exercise and a good pattern for exercise.

Lesson 4

Anger, Hostility, and Your Heart Rate

How does anger affect your heart rate? What are some strategies for controlling this anger in a healthy way?

Goals:

- To recognize that anger elevates the heart rate, sometimes to dangerous levels.
- To learn strategies to effectively and healthily deal with anger.

Key Concept:

Students can learn to control anger and to use heart energy efficiently.

Materials:

- One heart rate monitor (such as the Polar Vantage XL Heart Rate Monitor) for each student
- Exercise equipment
- Computer access
- One worksheet 4.1 for each student

Activity:

1. After students have put on their heart rate monitors, have them pair up.
2. Students will be exercising at five different stations. From each pair, select one of

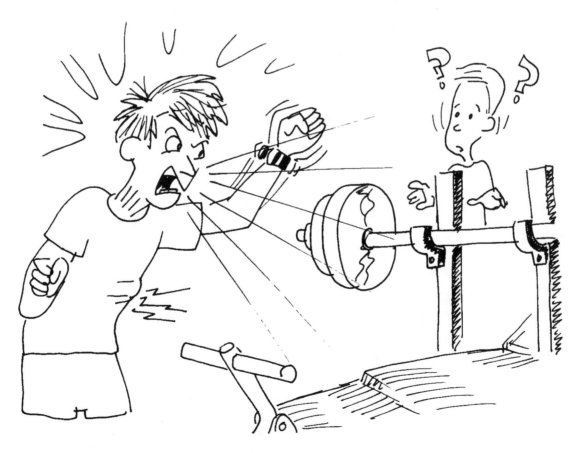

the students to scream at one of the machines for one minute at each station before he exercises at each of those stations. Have the other student simply exercise at each of the stations.

3. Have the screaming students push the red button on the Polar Vantage XL Heart Rate Monitor before and after screaming.
4. At the end of class, download the heart rate monitors and print out the results.
5. Have the pairs of students answer the questions on worksheet 4.1.

Teaching Tips:

So you don't lose control of the class, preface this activity by cautioning students to not get too carried away. Explain to students that heart rates reflect some emotions and that people can control emotions. Discuss why some people lose control of anger and how to prevent it through practicing staying calm, using heart rate monitors to demonstrate this. Give concrete suggestions for positive outlets for anger. Simple suggestions like counting to 10, taking deep breaths, closing your eyes, slowing your breathing, and so on. Discuss relaxation exercises. Discuss how exercise itself can alleviate stress or channel anger positively.

Notes

The Effects of Anger on Heart Rate

1. What were the differences in the heart rates of the two students at each exercise station?

2. Does anger increase or decrease heart rate?

3. What could happen to the heart rate if you were exercising and you also got angry?

4. Is anger helpful or harmful in exercise?

5. Consider situations when anger has escalated and affected performance of an athlete: angry at a basketball official and consequently thrown out of the game; tennis player angry at a call and has trouble focusing for the duration of the match; hockey player angry at another player and throws him against the wall and is ejected from the game. Would it help to practice staying calm?

6. What are some techniques you could use to practice staying calm and recording the information?

7. What are some situations in real life where staying calm is essential?

Lesson 5

Heart Rate Historical Geography

By converting the minutes to miles and using this information in a fun and entertaining way, students will understand that each day a person should exercise a minimum of 10 to 20 minutes, holding their heart rates in the target zone. The distance they actually cover is not as important as maintaining the heart rate in the target zone consistently while exercising.

Goal:

- To get students to focus on the fact that it is more important to exercise according to minutes in the target zone than according to the distance you run, bike, swim, or the like.

Key Concept:

Each student should understand that it is important to exercise holding their heart rates in the target zone for a set number of minutes, not how far they actually ran or biked.

Materials:

- One heart rate monitor for each student

Activity:

1. Using heart rate monitors, summarize each student's efforts each day according to heart rate information collected throughout the lesson in four ways: total minutes in the target zone, total minutes below the target zone, total minutes above the target zone, and average heart rate (table 4.1).
2. If you choose, using these totals, give students points each day, according to their personal efforts and individual fitness levels.
3. If you wish, you can convert the minutes to miles (for example, one minute equals 10 miles), having each student design a route across the United States and chart progress each day according to the minutes in the target zone. Goals could be set and periodically updated and recalculated.

Teaching Tips:

If possible, work with your students' regular classroom teachers to create interdisciplinary applications of heart rate monitor information. For example, students could pair up with one another and design a route that their combined efforts could reach. Each week, month, or nine weeks, new partners or squads could take another "Heart Rate Trip." You could design several variations of this activity, including the following:

Students could find another school on the Internet that uses heart rate monitors and work on heart rate routes and sites at which to collectively meet. Each week, students could record progress and figure new calculations, based on current results.

Students could also calculate distance "traveled" along unique landmarks, such as the Wall of China. History lessons could include facts about important landmarks along each route students have selected, including state capitals, large cities, Civil War battlefields, and so on.

You could also introduce mapping skills by "running" along interstate highways versus other roadways, determining the shortest route to a location, or racing across America.

TABLE 4.1   Sample Summary of Students' Efforts

Name	Average heart rate	Min. in target zone	Min. above target zone	Min. below target zone
Kim Wong	144 bpm	22	3	5
Lucia Albers	155 bpm	19	7	4
Beth Kruger	123 bpm	12	0	18
Simon Schultz	166 bpm	24	2	4

Multiply minutes in target zone by a constant so that the students advance across a map. The constant is determined by dividing the total distance traversed on the map by the number of days for the unit divided by the target zone minutes/day goal.

Lesson 6

Using Heart Rate to Understand the Principles of Fitness

In order to exercise the cardiovascular system effectively and safely it is important to know the three principles of fitness: progression of exercise—making sure you gradually build up the time and intensity of your exercise, overload—stressing the body with the right intensity to work the heart without overdoing it, and specificity—engaging in the exercise that is working the muscles and systems that you intend to shape up. By monitoring your heart rate, you can be sure you are safely and effectively exercising.

Goal:

- To learn how progression, overload, and specificity relate to cardiovascular fitness exercise programs.

Key Concepts:

By using heart rate as an indicator of effort and cardiovascular conditioning and by following directions, the student can receive credit for demonstrating the three principles of fitness.

Materials:

- Six stations for students to rotate through
- One heart rate monitor for each student
- Heart rate chart for each student (see table 4.2b)

Activity:

1. Assign all students to a specific beginning station. Have students rotate through each station two times. Allow students to stay at each station for two minutes.
2. The first time at each station, encourage students to hold their heart rates near the 140 range. (*Note*: Modify this target number for those individuals who have special needs.)
3. The second time at each station, encourage students to try to average about 10 beats per minute higher.

4. Have the students record their heart rates on a chart similar to the one shown in table 4.2a at each station before rotating to the next. Table 4.2b provides a blank chart for classroom use.
5. On each succeeding day of the activity, increase the time at each station by 30 seconds.

Teaching Tips:

Students should see that the increase in time or heart rate follows the principles of fitness.

Progression—gradually increase heart rate.
Overload—increasing time at each station shows this.
Specificity—*heart rate increase* is a specific result of effort when using the same equipment at each station.

TABLE 4.2a   Sample Heart Rate Chart for Station Use

Day 1	Min 1st	Min 2nd	Susan 1st	Susan 2nd	Tony 1st	Tony 2nd	Lee 1st	Lee 2nd	Jim 1st	Jim 2nd	June 1st	June 2nd
Station 1	140	155	140	150	140	163	135	155	123	145	133	144
Station 2	135	150	142	155	138	148	150	155	134	147	144	154
Station 3	140	149	135	148	134	144	140	150	139	149	137	148
Station 4	135	145	136	144	133	144	140	149	145	155	134	147
Station 5	141	151	135	146	125	140	134	146	144	156	141	164
Station 6	133	146	122	144	134	144	145	155	140	150	139	159

Demonstrating how heart rate is an indicator of effort and cardiovascular conditioning.

Notes

TABLE 4.2b   Heart Rate Chart for Classroom Use

Class period _____ Squad number ____ Sheet number ____ Grade level _____										
	Name	Name	Name	Name	Name	Name	Name	Name	Date	Total
Name										
HRM #										
HR AV										
In TZ										
–TZ										
+TZ										
HR AV										
In TZ										
–TZ										
+TZ										
HR AV										
In TZ										
–TZ										
+TZ										
HR AV										
In TZ										
–TZ										
+TZ										
HR AV										
In TZ										
–TZ										
+TZ										
HR AV										
In TZ										
–TZ										
+TZ										
HR AV										
In TZ										
–TZ										
+TZ										
		HRM Recording Chart for Each Squad								

Lesson 7

Heart Adventures Challenge Course

This integrated cross-curricular unit showcases all seven of the National Association of Sports and Physical Education (NASPE) national standards. See appendix B for a complete listing of these standards and other sample lessons to refer to for each standard.

Goals:

- To practice keeping the heart rate in the target zone throughout the entire challenge course.
- To learn about how the heart works.

Key Concepts:

In the Heart Adventures Challenge Course (on page 54), students move through a huge model of the heart, brain, and lungs, learning to understand and identify all areas and functions of the circulatory system. Train students to set up and disassemble the course, using the entire gymnasium. As students move through the course, they find themselves challenged by many basic forms of movement and different types of apparatus, using actions of pulling, throwing, catching, running, walking, crawling, climbing, jumping, and maneuvering. As a result, students following the course will take all their joints through their full ranges of motion, exercise in five basic postures, develop aerobic capacity individually and noncompetitively, use muscles in balancing activities, and experience endurance activities that will challenge muscles of the legs, stomach, arms, back, and chest. You can make competency assessments by stationing yourself at certain points and recording levels of proficiency in the categories we'll define.

The Heart Adventures Challenge Course educates students not only about the circulatory system but also which critical thinking, problem solving, and cooperative learning skills are necessary to successfully complete the course. In addition, students learn how these same skills are necessary both to meet the daily challenges in their lives and to improve their interactions with one another.

Materials:

- Heart Adventures Challenge Course
- Two to three adults
- A heart rate monitor for each student.

Activity:

1. Students enter the "Lifestyle Classroom" to find beautiful, larger-than-life equipment that encompasses the entire gymnasium. They soon discover they have just entered the heart and are standing in the middle of the right atrium.
2. As you invite them to walk through this color-coded obstacle course, students make their way through the giant mitral valve that is filling an archway with red balloons attached to it. As they look above, shiny red hoops hang high from the ceiling everywhere on the left side of the heart, and blue hoops hang low from the ceiling on the right side of the heart.
3. As students enter the left ventricle, they see ahead giant red doughnuts lining up for 20 feet, leading to long, matted red tunnels that branch in two directions.
4. Outside one of the branches of this aorta is a pathway that leads to the brain. There in the small fitness lab are three Nintendo power pads spread on the floor, hooked to color monitors. Students watch as their teachers challenge each other to move their feet faster on the padded mat so that their corresponding computer figure on the screen moves quicker that the other teacher's computer figure.

5. Leaving the brain, the students follow the path with you to the right atrium where they pick up a blue playground ball and a blue scooter board. Straight ahead lies a zigzagging blue mat maze.

6. Students on their own blue scooter board with their own blue playground ball wind through the tricuspid valve which is a blue archway filled with blue balloons. They toss their balls through each one of the hanging blue hoops.

7. As students wind through the right ventricle, they grab onto a blue rope that goes down the middle of the entire gymnasium through archways of blue balloons.

8. Using their arms to pull them down the pulmonary artery, they find themselves at the end of the ropes.

9. Leaving behind their blue scooter boards in the scooter board pit, they jump through a giant blue matted doughnut and spot colorful moonhoppers to bounce on the length of the lungs.

10. Having picked up oxygen (red playground ball) from the lungs and deposited carbon dioxide (blue playground ball) the students (red blood cells) leave going directly to the left atrium to begin the journey again.

11. The next day, have the students wear their heart rate monitors to record their heart rates while they are in the heart. Then have them take their printouts home to show their parents and invite them to the open house next week where the Heart Adventures Challenge Course will be set up for all to try.

Teaching Tips:

You can conduct health-related fitness tests using the Heart Adventures Challenge Course to identify how each area of fitness is needed in many everyday challenges as well as in high-energy activities. You can use the fitness assessments to educate students as to lifestyle fitness needs, based on their own lifestyle prescriptions. Polar Vantage XL Heart Rate Monitors provide the scientific information to ensure individualization of cardiovascular conditioning as well as provide documentation of effort and accountability based on each student doing his best.

Notes

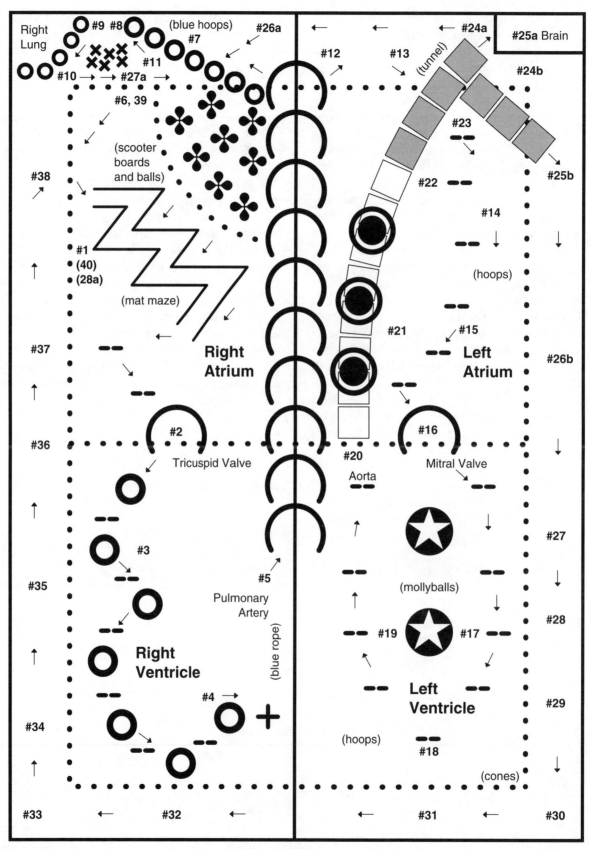

Lesson 8
Heartbeat Challenge

All students are equally able to meet this challenge from the heart, learning that effort and heart rate are personal responsibilities.

Goals:

- To use heart rate as the indicator of individual effort.
- To receive credit for maintaining an aerobic heart rate.

Key Concepts:

Students will learn what effort it takes each day for individual success in aerobic conditioning.

Materials:

- One heart rate monitor for each student

Activity:

1. For one week keep track of all the girls' average heart rates throughout physical education class as well as keep track of all the boys' average heart rates. Challenge the class to see who can maintain the highest average heart rate without going beyond the top limits of the aerobic target zone.
2. Take the 10 best days from each student and have the students average these to find out what their overall average heart rates were during their physical education classes.

3. Challenge the squads to see who maintains the best total average for one day of a unit. Reward the highest total average heart rate (don't give credit if the total is over the target zone), giving special recognition each week on the bulletin board.
4. Challenge different grades or classes to see which class maintains the highest average heart rate within the aerobic target zone for one class period or one week of classes.

Teaching Tips:

Find a school on the Internet that uses heart rate monitors. Challenge that school either by grade, by class, or by total physical education students to see which school maintains the highest average heart rates during physical education class for one week. Have each school document their results through charts or printouts. Using the minutes in the target zone, convert minutes to miles (one minute = 1 mile) and see how long it takes to meet that school at a location somewhere in the world. Have students recalculate results each week. For example, total minutes in the target zone for one school during physical education classes might be 2,000 minutes which could convert to 2,000 miles. If the meeting point for another school was 4,000 miles away, the other school would have to also accrue a total of 2,000 miles (minutes) to reach the projected meeting point. The next week, you could discuss a new destination and follow the same procedure. Maybe several schools worldwide could be involved!

Notes

Lesson 9

Charting Skill Proficiency

Using heart rate monitors, each student's heart rate can be recorded and can be the format of the physical education class itself.

Goals:

- To chart a student's skill learning with heart rate monitors
- To have students move toward competency and proficiency in movement forms

Key Concepts:

As the student's competency in a movement increases, less heart rate effort may be required for this movement. Thus, tracking the student's heart rate may help document the proficiency of the specific movement.

Materials:

- One heart rate monitor with downloading capabilities (such as the Polar Vantage XL Heart Rate Monitor) for each student
- Computer access

Activity:

1. Have each student perform a simple routine including several required movements.

This routine can be a dance, a specific basketball drill, or the like. Record the student's heart rate throughout the routine. Have the student press the store/recall button at each of the required movements.
2. Give each student a heart rate printout for the first time through the routine and another one for the final time through the routine.
3. Overlap the printout of the first routine with the printout of the final routine.
4. Note what the heart rate was at the markings for each of the required movements for the first time through the routine and the last time of the routine. Determine if the student was able to perform the required movements using less heart rate energy for the final time through the routine.
5. Determine if there was a difference in time between the required movements from the first time through as compared to the final time through the routine. Try to ascertain the reason for this (e.g., competency in many of the other movement forms).
6. Calculate what the average heart rates were throughout the routine for each student for the first time and for the final time. Was there a difference? Why?

Notes

Lesson 10

Heart Rate Solar Game

Travel through time and through space to reach your earthly heart fitness goals.

Goals:

- To use minutes in the target zone and average heart rate throughout class for moving through space.
- To keep students interested in achieving minutes in the target zone.

Key Concepts:

Students move throughout the solar system as they refresh their memories on where the planets are in relation to the earth. (At the elementary level, this is new information that may lend itself to an interdisciplinary approach.)

Materials:

- One heart rate monitor for each student
- Solar game board (see sample on page 58)

Activity:

1. Have each student wear a heart rate monitor throughout physical education class.

2. Each day for each student, record the minutes in the target zone, minutes above the target zone, minutes below the target zone, and average heart rate.
3. Using each student's average heart rate as the speed of the heart rate shuttle, move each student's shuttle the distance (miles) calculated by multiplying minutes in the target zone by the speed (average heart rate) for that person during physical education class (see table 4.3).
4. Allow students to select which planet they would like to start from and set goals, using the miles (minutes in target zone) multiplied by average heart rate minutes formula to orbit a planet and beam to the next planet.
5. For each planet visited, you may choose to reward students by allowing them to use special exercise equipment to travel on during the next orbit and so on.
6. Have students complete one orbit of each planet before beaming to the next planet.

Teaching Tips:

Try to work with the regular classroom teacher to tie this segment in with a science lesson.

TABLE 4.3   Sample Heart Rate Solar Game Calculations

Name	Average heart rate	Min. in target zone	Polar distance
Maria	145 bpm	20	2,900
Tom	150 bpm	15	2,250

Notes

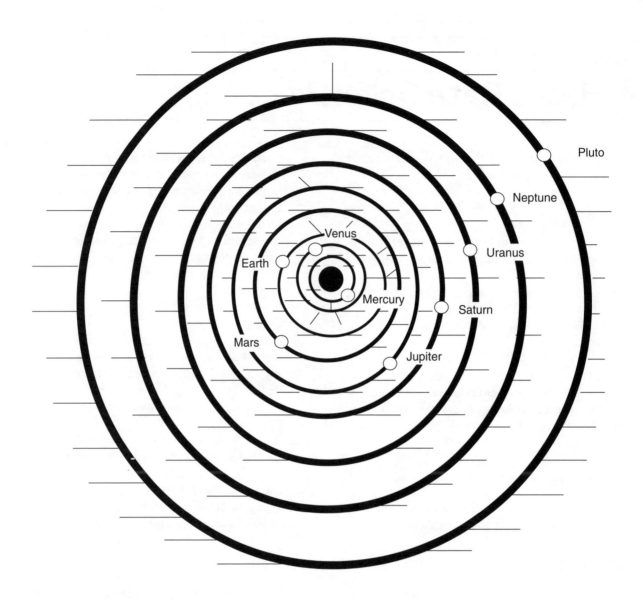

Lesson 11
Heart Rate Archery

By having students use their heart rate minutes in the target zone each day, we are getting them used to the idea that minutes in the target zone are always important and will be used for credit in each unit.

Goal:

- To use individual effort through heart rate minutes in the target zone for motivation using the heart rate archery game.

Key Concepts:

Using the heart rate monitor, students may see how many "arrows" of heart rate energy it takes to score a bull's-eye for heart healthy living and the real target—your healthy heart!

Materials:

- One target for each student (see sample on page 60)
- One heart rate monitor for each student

Activity:

1. For every 10 minutes the student holds her heart rate in the target heart rate zone, she may add one heart rate arrow to her "target."
2. Each arrow is worth 10 points.
3. To score a "Heart Healthy Bull's-Eye," a student must earn 10 arrows.
4. Challenge each student to score a bull's-eye every nine weeks.
5. Challenge each squad to combine arrows to challenge another squad.
6. Challenge the homerooms to see who has the most bull's-eyes per class.
7. See who has the most points: the teachers or the students (ratio of one teacher to one student).

Teaching Tips:

Consider collaborating with the students' art teacher to have each student make their own targets in art class.

Notes

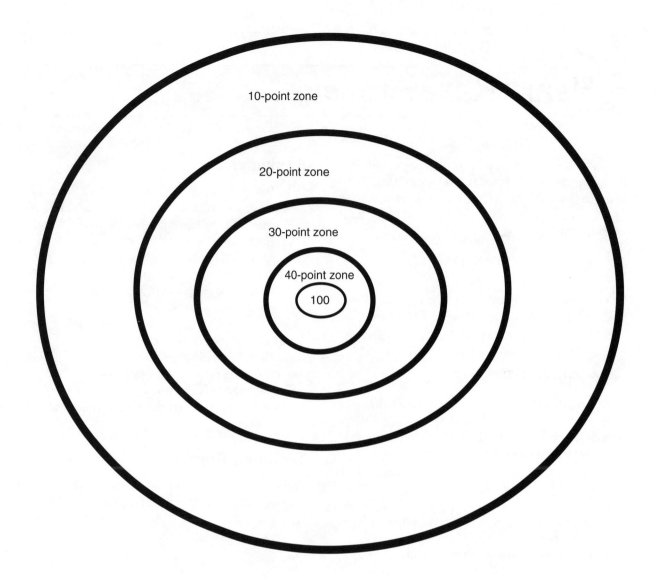

10-point zone

20-point zone

30-point zone

40-point zone

100

Intermediate
Lesson Plans

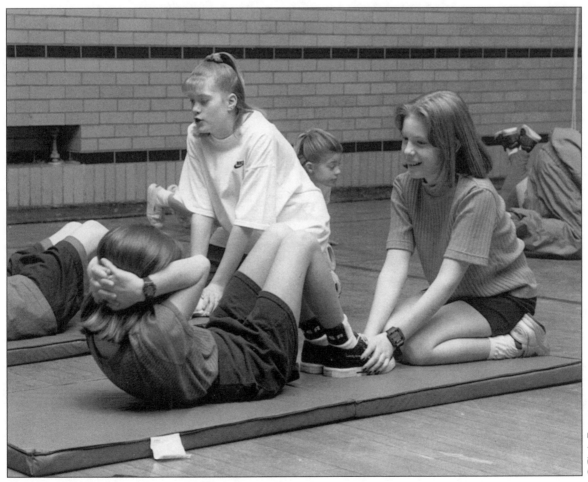

© Chris Brown

Students like to have choices in their lives (especially middle school and high school students). When it comes to exercise, nothing is greeted with more enthusiasm than giving students freedom to choose. Too often, however, students base their decisions on incomplete background information simply because of their age and limited experiences. Using heart rate monitors, you can give students healthy choices of how they may keep their heart rates in the target zone—as long as they understand that heart rates and responses to exercise are individual in nature. It is important that each middle school student recognizes that his exercise plan is his personal responsibility and that comparison to others is not the goal. Rather, the realistic goal is to improve on an individual basis as the result of making a personal investment in fitness.

Consequently, strive to make sure your students understand that their responsibility stops with their own bodies: Others in the class are not their responsibility. Help the student see the heart rate monitor as a "personal trainer" that keeps track of effort and improvement. Explain that this technology is a nonjudgmental entity that is objective and free from influences—either real or imagined in a student's mind. With this in mind, students are free to choose exercise equipment, never getting the answer to their fitness endeavors "wrong." Instead, appropriate heart rate during the exercise is the goal. Thus, whether a student chooses the exercise bike, the step machine, or the like, she can monitor her heart rate, providing both you and her with the documentation that many choices of exercise equipment are appropriate and that cardiovascular exercise requires consistent heart rates, no matter what type of equipment or exercise she selects each day. Perhaps even more importantly, students learn that they are all equal when it comes to effort and improvement. Indeed, through accurate heart rate monitoring, students will become fully aware that everyone is working at heart rates that are correct for them as individuals. Each student has the same responsibility to maintain correct heart rates throughout the exercise time whether the student is a boy or girl, athlete or nonathlete, well-conditioned or out-of-shape, physically challenged or not, and so on. Each person safely monitors heart rate throughout class for which she may earn credit for maintaining appropriate heart rates on an equal basis. Truly, appropriate use of heart rate monitors can "level the playing field." What better way to show students that exercise is a personal responsibility?

Lesson 1

Heart Rates and Conditioning Equipment

This lesson will help students apply how different intensities of a variety of exercises affect heart rates.

Goals:

- To be able to adjust intensity to stay within your target zone, depending on the activity.
- To understand that exercise equipment can be varied day to day or even during a workout as long as heart rate is maintained in the target heart rate zone.

- To understand that because heart rates are individual, it is each person's responsibility to maintain his own heart rate during exercise.

Key Concepts:

Heart rates are individual. Using conditioning equipment with adjustable intensity levels and a heart rate monitor to document successful personal effort, the exerciser can learn to rely on and benefit from continuous heart rate knowledge during exercise. Conditioning equipment varies

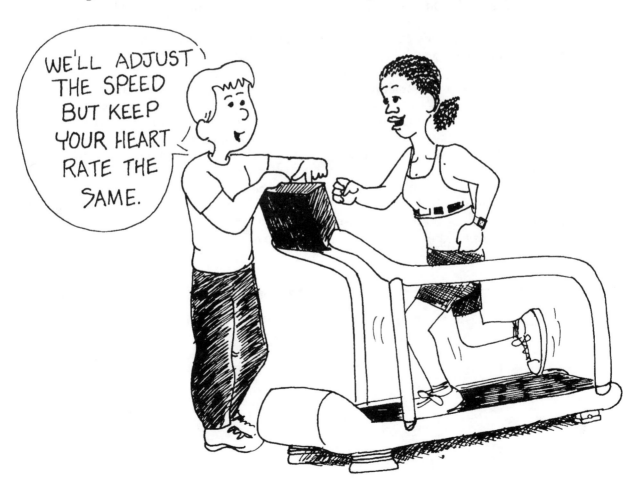

as to the type of intensity settings or adjustments that can be made by the student. Using heart rate monitors, each student can quickly adjust the intensity, according to her heart rate.

Materials:

- One heart rate monitor for each student
- Exercise equipment for five different stations (step machines, exercise bikes, ropes, running stairs, and the like)
- Heart rate chart for each squad or student (see table 4.2b)

Activity:

1. Have the students wear a heart rate monitor as they rotate through five different stations. Have students record their heart rates at the end of their exercise on a chart at each station.
2. Instruct the students that the goal is to exercise at the same heart rate for all five stations. The students should determine what heart rate each of them should strive to achieve. One way is to have them exercise in the individual target zone within 10 beats of 60 percent of maximum heart rate, which they can determine by subtracting their ages from 220 (see chapter 3, lesson 2). If you wish, award points to those individuals who maintained the same heart rate throughout all five stations (within 10 beats, plus or minus 10 beats).
3. At the beginning and end of each station, have each student push the store/recall button so that during the rotation, heart rates show recovery rates. You can have

students calculate their recovery rates as well.
4. Close the lesson by asking which exercise they liked best, which they liked least, and which station they would most likely do on their own.

Teaching Tips:

You can also demonstrate using two teachers how the same resistance setting on one exercise bike produces two completely different heart rates as recorded by the heart rate monitor each is wearing.

Have as wide a variety of equipment as possible. Here are some ways to borrow or buy more equipment. Try or adapt them to suit your needs and think up your own ideas as well! (See also appendix C for fund-raising ideas.) Ask local fitness equipment dealers to loan the school equipment for a two-week period. Use the equipment and station routine for an open house, inviting parents to participate if possible. To convince local fitness equipment dealers to help you, tell them that this can be an open house for displaying their products. After all, everyone likes free, positive advertising! In this way, everyone benefits: Your students will be exposed to a wide variety of equipment, and the dealers will be showing their goods to the entire community.

Hold a fund-raiser in which parents and community members try to guess what their heart rates are as they try each station: Cover the heart rate monitors with wristbands, and when the parents try to guess, see how close they are. For each beat they are off, they contribute a certain amount of money (in cents). For each time they guess correctly they receive a certain amount of money (in cents).

Notes

Lesson 2

Smoking and Heart Rate

Recently, use of tobacco by children under the age of 18 has increased dramatically. This lesson helps children understand how smoking directly affects their hearts.

Goals:

- To alert students to the fact that smoking is hazardous to cardiovascular health because it robs the heart of oxygen, constricts blood vessels, and otherwise does harm, which often is reflected in heart rates that are higher for smokers than nonsmokers.
- To present objective heart rate data showing the effects of tobacco use on the heart rate.

Key Concepts:

Smoking increases the heart rate because nicotine is classified as a stimulant.

Smoking constricts blood vessels, also causing higher heart rates, indicating poor cardiovascular fitness.

Materials:

- Five adult smokers (who volunteer)
- Five adult nonsmokers
- One or more heart rate monitors (such as Polar Accurex II Heart Rate Monitor)

Activity:

1. Place the heart rate monitor on each of the 10 adults and record each adult's heart rate each minute for five minutes as they sit.
2. Find the average of the heart rates recorded for each person. Then average the heart rates of the smokers and the nonsmokers.
3. Ask "What is the difference in heart rate at rest for the smokers compared to the nonsmokers?"
4. Now calculate the difference over the course of 10 years for a nonsmoker's resting heart rate of 75 beats per minute and a smoker's heart rate of 95 beats per minute: (95 beats × 60 min. × 24 hr. × 365 days × 10 yr.) – (75 beats × 60 min. × 24 hr. × 365 days × 10 yr.) = _____.

Teaching Tips:

Higher resting heart rates can be one indication that the person's cardiovascular fitness is not as good as it could be. This is because the heart is not as efficient with each beat of the heart and is unable to pump as much volume per beat. In addition, higher resting heart rates mean that the heart does not have as much time to rest in between beats.

Notes

Lesson 3
Caffeine and Heart Rate

Caffeine increases the heart rate because it is a stimulant.

Goals:

- To alert students to the effects on heart rate of using caffeine on a day-to-day basis through the consumption of pop and chocolates.
- To alert students that they can choose noncaffeinated pops that do not elevate heart rates.

Key Concepts:

Students will explore the questions "Can the short-term effects of consuming caffeinated soda be differentiated as far as resting heart rates?" and "Can the long-term effects on resting heart rate of consuming caffeinated soda be predicted?"

Materials:

- One heart rate monitor for each student
- One worksheet 5.1 for each student

Activity:

1. Place the heart rate monitor on each student for five minutes while they are sitting. Find and record the class's average heart rate for each student.
2. Ask the students to separate into three groups:
   a. Those who do not drink any caffeinated soda each day
   b. Those who drink one to three cans of caffeinated soda each day
   c. Those who drink four or more cans of caffeinated soda each day
3. Find the average resting heart rate for each of the three groups.
4. Have the students complete worksheet 5.1.

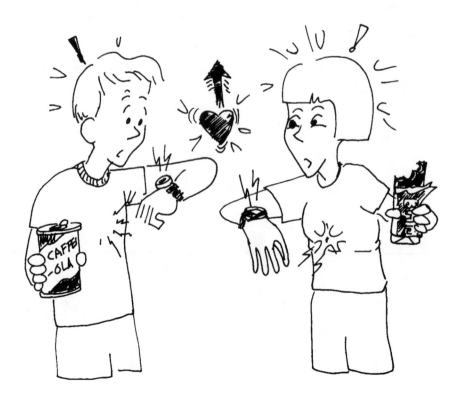

1. What were the differences among the three groups?

2. Which group had the highest average heart rate?

3. Which group had the lowest average heart rate?

4. What do you think crack, cocaine, methamphetamines, and heroin do to the heart rate and to the risk of heart disease?

5. Explain how this contributes to our costs for medical and life insurance. What can you do to stop the use of harmful drugs?

Lesson 4

Gifts From the Heart

Excellent cardiovascular fitness results in extra energy for living. Students have choices of how to use this energy as "gifts" from the heart by helping out someone in the community.

Goals:

- To show how better cardiovascular fitness may improve the energy levels of individuals.
- To get students thinking about investing this energy back into the community as individuals helping individuals.

Key Concepts:

The heart rate printouts from heart rate monitors can reflect heart rate evidence of a fitness routine, exercise time, or, in this case, of heart rate energy "given" to help someone in the community. Think of the impact on our country if we, as teachers, can motivate our students to invest their extra heart energy into our communities! Let's spread the idea of "giving" heart rate energy, school by school and state by state.

Materials:

- One heart rate monitor with downloading capabilities (such as the Polar Vantage XL Heart Rate Monitor) for each student
- Computer access

Activity:

1. For extra credit, students can check out heart rate monitors during the school day (perhaps during study hall) or during a scheduled after-school "gifts from the heart" time.
2. Students wear the monitor while engaging in an activity that shows kindness of their choice. Some suggestions include the following:
   - Raking an elderly person's lawn
   - Helping someone who is disabled with a chore
   - Volunteering at a daycare center
   - Working at the school, helping the custodians
   - Volunteering at the local humane society
   - Helping deliver Meals on Wheels to the elderly
   - Shoveling snow for a neighbor
   - Volunteering to help at a local hospital
   - Babysitting for a neighbor at no charge
   - Spending one hour cleaning a park
   - Cleaning graffiti off one wall in your city
3. Students record their heart rates throughout the activity.
4. Students return their heart rate monitors, download the information into the computer, and receive a graphic printout of their gifts of kindness. Have them analyze the average heart rate, the total heartbeats, and determine investment versus the return in this project (which is calculated by the computer program from the downloaded data).

Teaching Tips:

Students receive 10 points for each gift from the heart with no limit on the number of gifts throughout the year. Use one wall in the gym to attach each printout of each student's "gift from the heart." Challenge the students to fill the wall with the school's "gifts from the heart." Contact your local media to bring positive attention to your students' efforts and to spread the idea to other schools.

Lesson 5

Social Studies and Cardiovascular Fitness

This interdisciplinary lesson encourages students to research using a library or Internet access and to apply what they've learned about heart rate.

Goals:

- To alert students to the fact that cardiovascular diseases are detrimental to the health of citizens of other countries as well as our own.
- To brainstorm a list of factors that may influence the rates of cardiovascular disease, country by country.

Key Concepts:

Industrialized countries have the highest incidences of heart disease, costing the world untold billions. Having the students conduct this research may create interest in others worldwide (perhaps through the Internet). Indeed, prevention can be our greatest investment in this global concern. Discussion of the factors present in the lifestyles of the countries should result in students looking at their own lifestyles when making decisions now and in the future.

Materials:

- Library
- Internet access (optional)
- A heart rate monitor for each student
- One worksheet 5.2 for each student

Activity:

1. Have each student choose a different country to write a report about describing the three leading causes of death in that country.
2. Have them answer the following questions in their reports:
   - Does the information list cardiovascular-related deaths as one of the top three killers in the country?
   - What is the projected cost to the country each year as a result of cardiovascular illness?
   - Do more heart attacks and cardiovascular-related illnesses occur in the more-industrialized countries or in the less-industrialized countries?
3. Have each student wear a heart rate monitor and record the heart rate after each of the activities below:
A.
   - Pretend to take a pizza out of a freezer and put it in the oven.
   - Remove the pizza and pretend to sit down and eat it.
B.
   - Run after another student who is pretending to be a rabbit.
   - After being chased for 10 minutes, the rabbit allows himself to be caught.
4. Have each student complete worksheet 5.2.

Notes

1. What was the difference in heart rate energy in a country where the citizens simply eat food and do not have to hunt or gather food?

2. What are the effects of years of eating food readily available versus years of eating food you have had to hunt or gather?

3. Write a paragraph about the importance of exercise in the industrialized countries and how heart disease illnesses could be affected by this.

Lesson 6

Critical Thinking and Writing About Heart Rate Information

This interdisciplinary exercise asks students to communicate what they've learned about applying heart rate information to exercise.

Goals:

- To demonstrate knowledge of heart rate printouts by explaining the meaning of various terms as they pertain to one of a student's own printouts.
- To encourage parents to be more interested in their child's explanation of her own printout.

Key Concepts:

Each student is given a heart rate graph printout which contains the same basic information, looking at target heart rate zone, maximum heart rate, resting heart rate, recovery heart rate, and so on. The students will be asked to write about their printout, but the explanations from students will be possibly quite varied. For example, a student may explain that her heart rate was not in the target zone during the activity portion because the teams were too large or that there was not enough equipment. Or a student may explain that her heart rate was always in the target zone during an activity because the activity was so interesting and fun, perhaps a favorite. Use this as an opportunity for students to express their emotional and social thoughts about physical education and fitness activities in general. This could lead to discussions on what activities the students intend to use following the school year and what physical education activities have influenced the students' predictions of future activities.

Materials:

- One heart rate monitor with downloading capabilities (such as the Polar Vantage XL Heart Rate Monitor) for each student
- Computer access
- Printouts from Polar Vantage XL Heart Rate Monitors

Activity:

1. Using a graph (see example paragraph on page 72), have each student write a paragraph explaining her heart rate information to a parent.
2. Make sure students use the following words in the paragraph: warm-up, target heart rate zone, maximum heart rate, resting heart rate, recovery heart rate, minutes in the target heart rate zone, activity, cooldown, heart rate, markers at bottom of graph, and solid horizontal line.

Teaching Tips:

Have the students write how they enjoyed the activity part of the class and if that is reflected in the heart rate printout. Ask the students to suggest how the heart rates might be improved if the activity segment showed heart rates too low or too high.

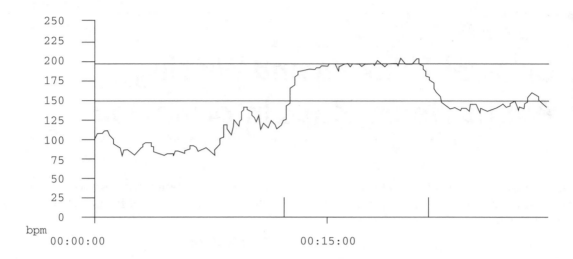

The first part of the graph shows that my resting heart rate was in the low 80s. My maximum heart rate which equals 208 is figured by taking 220 and subtracting my age. The two solid lines that go horizontally are the upper limits of my aerobic zone or target heart rate zone. This was figured by taking my maximum heart rate and multiplying it by 70% and again by 85%. My target heart rate zone is about 150 to 190 beats per minute. The heart rate monitor was set for my target zone so that if I was not in the aerobic zone, the heart rate monitor would beep at me. This helped me keep the correct pace while I was exercising.

The printout you see above is from my physical education class showing that I did my personal best throughout the aerobic time of class.

The markers on the bottom line of the graph show that I pushed the correct button on the heart rate monitor to show when I began the running time and when I ended the running time. My teacher said that by having the heart rate monitors, we all would be able to receive credit for doing our best. When we finished the running time, notice how my heart rate recovered to below the aerobic zone. We always continue to move following the areobic time because a good cool-down is important for safe exercise. Following the cool-down, I participated in volleyball. My heart rate was in the 140s which is aerobic. This shows that I was giving a good effort during the activity portion of class and that the activity of volleyball helped to condition my heart.

Notes

Lesson 7

Math and Science—Using the Karvonen Formula

Note: Students should first find their resting heart rates (see chapter 3, lesson 1) before completing this lesson.

We all need to understand that not every person's target heart rate zone is figured exactly the same way. This cannot be reinforced enough. For a generalized heart rate zone the commonly used formula of 220 minus age multiplied by 70 percent (.70) and 85 percent (.85) works fairly well. The range of this zone is wide enough that most individuals will find a comfort zone. However, for those who are in the high or low end of cardiovascular fitness, you may have to help them modify these zones somewhat. Because the heart rate monitors provide an accurate, continuous reading of the heart rate, it is feasible to compute the correct heart rate zone as accurately as is possible. We encourage you to tap into this technology because the more careful and exact at figuring the target heart rate zone we can be, the better. The Karvonen formula is unique as target heart rate zone formulas go because in addition to figuring in an individual's age, it figures in the individual's resting heart rate. This lesson helps students understand the process of calculating a target zone by taking a closer look at how to individualize a target heart rate zone.

Goal:

- To be able to use the Karvonen formula to figure the individual target heart rate zone.

Key Concepts:

Students must find the average of their resting heart rates taken six days in a row to determine readings that are as accurate as possible. The best time to find the true resting heart rate is when you wake up in the morning, before you have even raised your head from the pillow.

Materials:

- Pen and paper
- Calculators
- One heart rate monitor for each student (could be worn all night to determine the most accurate resting heart rate)
- One worksheet 5.3 for each student

Activity:

Hand out worksheet 5.3 in class and have (or help) students fill it out.

Teaching Tips:

Using the heart rate monitor, have students find their pulses as they sit in class. Have them record this and see if they find a difference between the readings they found first thing each morning and in class. Ask "What is the difference if you wear a heart rate monitor all night? What was the lowest reading?" Discuss the accuracy of heart rate monitors as well as the difference between the first pulse taken in the morning and one taken while sitting in class.

Using the Karvonen Formula to Figure Your Target Heart Rate

One way to find your target heart rate is to use the Karvonen formula. The usual formula of starting with 220 minus age does not take into account those individuals who vary greatly from the average. For example, if you are in terrific cardiovascular condition, your resting heart rate could be much lower than someone in the same age bracket as you. The Karvonen formula takes this into account, allowing you to individualize your target heart rate zone by using the resting heart rate as another variable. (Remember, you can calculate your resting heart rate—the lowest number of beats per minute your heart contracts at rest—by checking your pulse as soon as you wake up in the morning, before you lift your head from the pillow.) Generally a person with a very low resting heart rate may have a target zone that is 10 to 20 beats lower than a person with a high resting heart rate, for example, 130 to 170 versus 140 to 180.

1. Find your maximum heart rate by subtracting your age from 220: 220 – _____ = _____.
2. Write your resting heart rate here: _____.
3. Subtract your resting heart rate (line 2) from your maximum heart rate (line 1).
4. Multiply the answer to line 3 by .60 (60% of line 3) = _____.
5. Add your resting heart rate (line 2) to line 4: _____.
6. This total is the minimum heart rate you should maintain during the aerobic segment of your workout. Enter this number as the lower limit of your target zone on your heart rate monitor.
7. Now write your maximum heart rate here (the answer to line 1): _____.
8. Write your resting heart rate from line 2: _____.
9. Subtract your resting heart rate (line 8) from your maximum heart rate (line 7): _____.
10. Multiply line 9 by .80 (80% of line 9): _____.
11. Add the resting heart rate (line 8) to line 10: _____.
12. This total is the maximum heart rate you should maintain during the aerobic segment of your workout. Enter this number as the upper limit of your target zone on your heart rate monitor.

Keep your heart rate between your upper and lower limits (_____ and _____) to gain aerobic benefits!

Lesson 8

Environment and Heart Rate— Energy Too Precious to Waste

This lesson helps students quantify the amount of energy wasted in terms of heartbeats when we have to pick up after one another.

Goal:

- To show that when each one of us disregards the need to pick up after ourselves on the Earth, energy is both wasted while we discard something and while people retrieve our garbage.

Key Concepts:

Heart rate energy needed to clean up after ourselves is more efficient than the heart rate energy needed of one person cleaning up after many. Measuring this using heart rate information during the activity should bring objective documentation to this concept.

Materials:

- Enough balls of varying sizes for each student to have one
- One heart rate monitor for each student
- Plastic garbage container or any container in which to place balls

Activity:

1. With all students wearing heart rate monitors, have each student throw a ball (of any size) anywhere in the gym. This is to simulate throwing garbage of some type away during the day (e.g., pop cans, paper, and the like).
2. Have the students push the store/recall button when they throw the ball down and push it again when they are finished throwing (this should be almost immediate).
3. Select one student to pick up all the equipment that was thrown down by all the students, using a plastic garbage container to gather all the different types of balls or other equipment used. Encourage the student to pick up as fast as possible.
4. Have that student push the store/recall button when she begins the task of gathering all the thrown-away equipment, then again when she is finished gathering all the equipment.
5. For those students wearing Polar Vantage XL Heart Rate Monitors, print out the heart rates of all the students and of the one student that gathered all the equipment. Record the average heart rates for those students wearing the Polar Accurex II Heart Rate Monitor and compare the average heart rates between the one student who gathered equipment and those who simply threw the equipment away.
6. Discuss what heart rate energy was used by the student who gathered compared to the heart rate energy of all the other throwing students combined.
7. Discuss the heart rate energy used to clean up after others in our society.
8. Do the activity again, except this time record each student picking up the ball he threw away. Ask "What was the heart energy when all were cleaning up after themselves as compared to when one person did all the work alone?"

Teaching Tips:

You could vary the activity by using real garbage, having students separate it into cans, plastic, newspapers, and so on. Consider organizing a community cleanup or recycling day, having all volunteers wear heart rate monitors.

Lesson 9

Harnessing Heart Rate Energy and Improving Your Health

Exercise the heart and help the environment at the same time!

Goal:

- To alert students to the fact that investing in cardiovascular fitness can also be a productive investment in saving our environment.

Key Concepts:

Cardiovascular exercise means elevating the heart rate. Of course, we can do this many different ways. The key is to know your heart rate throughout a workout. This knowledge allows you to exercise in the most efficient and safe way. But beyond the personal gain of cardiovascular fitness, students will consider the idea of harnessing their heart rate energy by turning it into useful endeavors that help the environment. People power, after all, is a much cleaner option than burning coal!

Materials:

- One heart rate monitor with downloading capabilities (such as the Polar Vantage XL Heart Rate Monitor) for each student
- Equipment for several stations
- Computer access

Activity:

1. Each day have students hold their heart rates in the target zone for 10 minutes during physical education class. Offer students several choices of activity: running, using exercise equipment, jumping rope, and the like.
2. Document the 10 minutes in the target zone using printouts from the Polar Vantage XL HRM or by recording data on a chart for the Polar Accurex II HRM. Record this information in each student's portfolio.
3. Discuss what would happen if while performing all activities they were hooked up to generators that transformed their heart energy into electricity. Discuss the benefits to society if everyone, everyday used exercise equipment that also generated electricity, using it safely by holding their heart rates in the target heart rate zones for at least 20 minutes each day. Discuss the possible benefits to our health, our families, our productivity in jobs, our combined heart power to Earth power (collective individual energy to work potential), our self-esteems, our joint efforts, our feelings of working for the good of humankind, and our use of a renewable source of energy.
4. Have students work on an art project in which they design machines to harness the heart power generated by people.

Teaching Tips:

You may wish to have students form groups or teams, placing one member of each team at each station. Challenge other teams to see if all team members can contribute 9 to 10 minutes of exercise in the target zone. Have team members switch stations (or switch stations and organize new team groupings) and then challenge another team. Award points to "build" something as a class or school project using their energy (e.g., a road, castle, or pyramid).

Remind students that their real responsibility is to keep their heart rates at the correct level for them. All of us should feel comfortable working out when we are truly doing our personal bests. Encourage students to think about which exercise station or equipment they liked best. Emphasize that as long as an activity is safe and good for you it is worthwhile.

Lesson 10

Banking on Your Heart Rate

Use physical education class to teach students to invest in themselves physically, mentally, and emotionally. In this activity, students learn to think about investing in personal fitness, which they accumulate through regular heart rate deposits.

Goals:

- To learn that investing is worthwhile, whether talking about aerobic benefits, financial benefits, or the like.
- To focus on cardiovascular fitness, using minutes in the target zone versus miles in the target zone.

Key Concepts:

Heart rate monitors can provide the individualization, immediate feedback, and documentation to show that fitness is cumulative and that each of us must make regular "deposits" to see good "returns." In this heart rate monitor activity, students can turn minutes invested in aerobic fitness into heart rate dollars. Teach students how to invest in their cardiovascular fitness and understand interest rates using their heart rates. Not only will they learn to think about their investments in personal fitness, they'll learn a little money math, too!

Materials:

- One heart rate monitor for each student
- Calculators

Activity:

1. During each physical education class, record average heart rate, minutes in the target zone, minutes below the target zone, and minutes above the target zone for each student.

2. Each day, have each student deposit her heart rate dollars in the bank, using her average heart rate as the amount of heart rate dollars. Multiply the heart rate bank account total by the interest rate percentage, which is the minutes in the target zone for that day. Explain that interest rates vary from student to student as in the real world of banking.

3. For example, Min's average heart rate is 145 and her minutes in the target zone are 15. The addition of 145 brings her total in heart rate dollars to $1,000.00. So she multiplies $1,000.00 by 15 percent (.15), which equals $150.00. Min adds $150.00 to her heart rate account, bringing her total to $1,150.00. Her minutes out of the target zone are withdrawals against her account (which are calculated after the deposit of the minutes in the target zone). If Min's minutes out of the target zone are 5, she would multiply the balance of $1,150.00 by 5 percent (.05), which is $57.50. Min then subtracts $57.50 from $1,150.00, which leaves her with $1,092.50.

Teaching Tips:

Devise a system in which heart rate dollars can be converted to special prizes at the end of each month, quarter, or school year! Students then can "shop" and "spend" their "money." Find sponsorships from community businesses to donate special prizes, targeting those who have a direct interest in students getting and staying fit (e.g., shoe stores, fitness stores, hospitals, insurance companies, and the like).

Advanced Lesson Plans

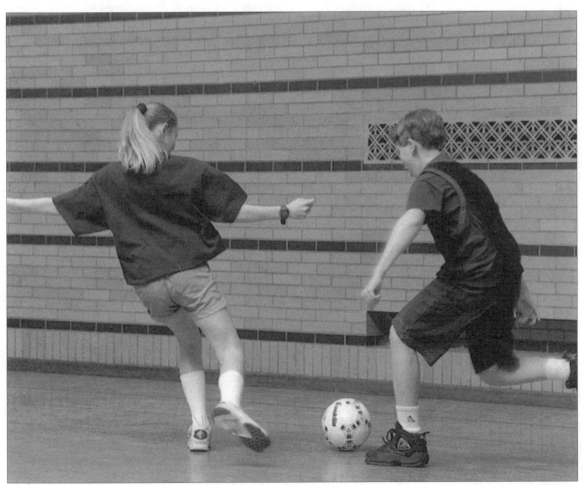

© Chris Brown

Often for older or more advanced students, you can individualize cardiovascular conditioning to increase motivation. For example, when using heart rate monitors, you can give students choices as to what type of cardiovascular workout they want to work on each day. Students who learn how to figure the different heart rate zones and what they are used for are more likely to take a more personalized approach to their own programs. Thus, they learn to choose the type of exercise that suits their needs, knowing that they'll receive credit from the instructor for their daily successes in meeting their goals. They will also learn valuable lifestyle lessons to apply to their private lives independently.

Lesson 1

Heart Rate Zones and Personalizing Your Training

Students can learn how to compute their heart rate zones as well as how to monitor themselves day to day.

Goals:

- To select and demonstrate successful cardiovascular conditioning during each physical education class
- To use different exercises or equipment while still exercising in their individual heart rate zones
- To understand how different factors can affect performance (e.g., heat, humidity)

Key Concepts:

As the heart rate monitors give students daily feedback, they will begin to notice patterns of how various factors can cause their heart rates to go above or below their zones (e.g., heat, humidity, and anxiety all increase heart rate). By using heart rate monitors, students can adjust their training approaches continuously, thereby maintaining training effects.

Materials:

- One heart rate monitor for each student
- One worksheet 6.1 for each student
- Calculators (optional)

Activity:

1. See chapter 3, lesson 2 for determining target heart rate zones under "Activity" heading.
2. Have students complete worksheet 6.1.

Notes

Determine your target heart rates for the five heart rate zones in table 6.1. Remember: Your maximum heart rate is determined by 220 – (your age).

1. Moderate activity zone (50 to 60% HRmax): _____ bpm to _____ bpm
2. Weight management zone (60 to 70% HRmax): _____ bpm to _____ bpm
3. Aerobic zone (70 to 80% HRmax): _____ bpm to _____ bpm
4. Anaerobic threshold zone (80 to 90% HRmax): _____ bpm to _____ bpm
5. Red-line zone (90 to 100% HRmax): _____ bpm to _____ bpm

TABLE 6.1   The Five Training Heart Rate Zones and Their Uses

Heart rate zone	% HRmax	Workout duration	System trained	Why use this HR zone?	Term for this zone
Moderate activity	50 to 60	60+ min.	Metabolic fuel burn	Burns fat slowly	Easy pace
Weight management	60 to 70	30+ min.	Cardiorespiratory	Burns fat faster	Base work
Aerobic	70 to 80	8 to 30 min.	Aerobic	Burns fat fastest	Long-term
Anaerobic	80 to 90	5 to 8 min.	Lactate clearance	Builds muscle	Tempo
Red-line	90 to 100	1 to 5 min.	Anaerobic	Builds muscle	Short-term

Lesson 2

Heart Rates and Conditioning Equipment

Students each wear a heart rate monitor as they rotate through five different stations during physical education class. Students record their heart rates on a chart at each station. Knowing the heart rate is the key to determining what exercise is right for your heart (which one meets your needs).

Goals:

- To determine individual heart rate target zones.
- To exercise at the same heart rate at all five stations.

Key Concepts:

Because all stations can be aerobic, depending on the effort the student makes, it becomes clear to students that they can base their choices of exercise on individual preference. For the exercise to be beneficial to the heart, however, they must closely monitor themselves to ensure that they are staying in their individual target heart rate zones.

Materials:

- One heart rate monitor (such as the Polar Accurex II Heart Rate Monitor) for each student
- Five stations (e.g., exercise bikes, step machines, rowing machines, jump ropes, cross-country ski machines, step benches, slideboards, and the like)
- A chart by each station for each student. The students can write their own names as they arrive, saving the teacher's limited prep time.
- Pencils

Activity:

1. After students put on their heart rate monitors, have each determine what heart rate she is striving to achieve. You may, for example, suggest that students exercise within 10 beats of 60 percent of the maximum heart rate.
2. Instruct each student to press the store/recall button at the beginning and at the end of each station so that during the rotation, heart rates show recovery, dropping from the exercise heart rate to heart rates that are at least 30 beats lower. In other words, allow a cool-down between stations, perhaps by walking slowly and stretching between stations.
3. You may wish to award points to individuals who maintain the same heart rate throughout all five stations (within plus or minus 10 beats).
4. Close the session by asking which exercise the students liked best, which they liked least, and which station they would most likely do on their own.

Lesson 3

Heart Rates and Anaerobic Conditioning

When students run short sprints as fast as they can, they typically run out of breath. This is because the heart cannot circulate enough oxygen fast enough for the person to continue. But, by allowing for a brief recovery time, depending on how high the intensity and how long the individual ran, the body will rebound, and the student will be able to begin another short sprint. The time it takes to gather enough oxygen and to circulate it fast enough to keep the student running is called the heart rate recovery time, after which the student can once again sprint. Using a heart rate monitor with downloading capabilities, such as the Polar Vantage XL Heart Rate Monitor, you or the student can plot the high heart rates and the low heart rates to determine when the sprinter is in the anaerobic limit and when the sprinter has recovered sufficiently to begin another sprint.

Goals:

- To be able to read a graph that shows two different individuals running the same series of sprints and to recognize the vast differences the same set of sprints had on the individuals.
- To understand that sprints require heart rates to recover and that the recovery time may well vary from individual to individual, depending on many factors, including cardiovascular conditioning, stress, medications, asthma, weather, humidity, and so on.

Key Concepts:

Using heart rate as an indicator of recovery, the heart rate monitor allows for individualized anaerobic conditioning. But without close monitoring, individuals may be training at levels that are not effective and quite possibly unsafe.

Materials:

- One heart rate monitor with downloading capabilities (such as the Polar Vantage XL Heart Rate Monitor) for each student
- Computer access
- One worksheet 6.2 for each student

Activity:

1. Have students run for 100 yards holding their heart rates at the 190- to 200-beat range (middle school age target zone).
2. When their heart rates have dropped 40 beats, have them run another 100 yards in the 190- to 200-beat range.
3. Repeat this a total of four times and download the results.
4. Evaluate the printouts to see if each student followed directions.
5. Note the differences among students in the number of seconds they had to wait for heart rates to drop 40 beats.
6. Between each of the four 100-yard sprints, can you see differences in the number of seconds spent waiting for the heart rates to drop each time or were they all the same?

Teaching Tips:

Make sure students are aware that only their heart rates are of concern in this activity. Discourage students from making comparisons based on the individual times of each 100-yard sprint; instead, emphasize using their heart rates as the correct pacing. Students will begin running 100-yard sprints and doing stretches at various starting and stopping points around the track. Each student should be given an individualized agenda, thus avoiding observations by others and comparisons with others which can discourage those with lower fitness levels. Have the students try running with the wind and then against the wind to see if they can detect differences in heart rate responses.

Look at the two graphs below (figure 6.1, *a* and *b*) depicting two different students running the same series of seven 200-meter sprints, six 100-meter sprints, and six 50-meter sprints.

1. Did each athlete recover sufficiently after each sprint in each set?
2. If you were a teacher or coach, how would you design an anaerobic workout that was right for each individual?

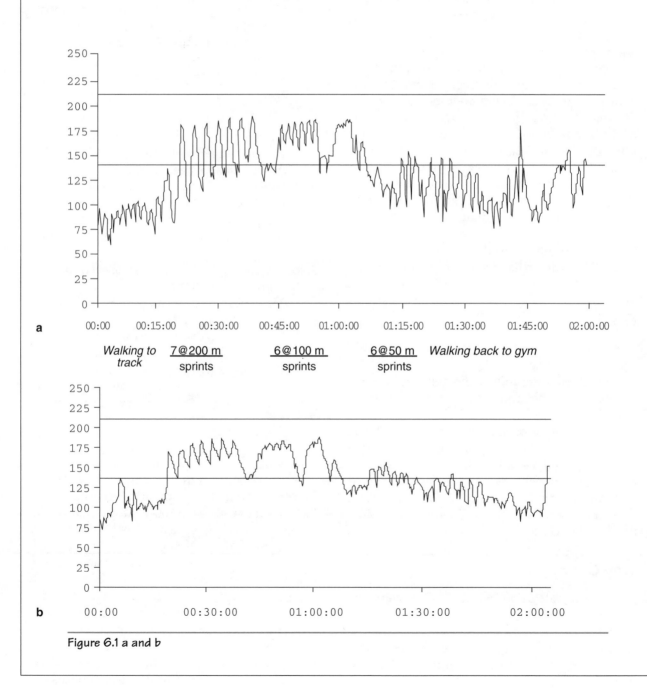

a

Walking to track   <u>7 @ 200 m</u> sprints   <u>6 @ 100 m</u> sprints   <u>6 @ 50 m</u> sprints   *Walking back to gym*

b

Figure 6.1 a and b

Lesson 4

Using Heart Rate Monitors in Speech Class

This interdisciplinary lesson allows students to track how anxiety and stress can affect their heart rates.

Goal:

- To understand that heart rates may reflect anxiety, anger, stress, and the like, and that people can learn to control these emotions.

Key Concepts:

Heart rate monitors aren't only for physical education! Finding out what causes anxiety and how to control it is important in many jobs. Of course, different jobs suit different people. For example, some people are better suited to doing jobs that do not require public speaking, deadlines, being in front of the camera, life and death decision making, or other forms of high pressure. Giving a speech is something that generally causes anxiety, but can be practiced and is not life-threatening. Finding out how to control stress using heart rate as one indicator is a fun activity that can help students learn about relaxation, focus, courage, and preparation.

Materials:

- One heart rate monitor with downloading capabilities (such as the Polar Vantage XL Heart Rate Monitor) for every student giving a speech
- One worksheet 6.3 for each student giving a speech

Activity:

1. Have each speechmaker wear a heart rate monitor throughout the entire class period.
2. Have each speechmaker record her heart rate throughout the class period.
3. When it is time for a student to deliver her speech, have her push the store/recall button.
4. Have each speechmaker keep the heart rate monitor on for the rest of the class period, having everyone stop recording at the end of the class period.
5. You or each student downloads the heart rate information into the computer.
6. Give the students the printouts of their heart rates and have them complete worksheet 6.3.

--- *Notes* ---

1. What was your average heart rate during your speech?
2. What was your highest heart rate during your speech?
3. What was your lowest heart rate during your speech?
4. How long did it take for your heart rate to recover to the average heart rate you had before you gave the speech?
5. Based on your heart rate information, do you think heart rate and anxiety are closely related? Why or why not?

6. Name some careers in which it is important to be able to keep anxiety under control.

7. Can you slow your heart rate by trying to relax?
8. What happens when your heart rate speeds up even though you are not exercising?

9. How do you feel when this happens?

10. What are some practices that help you control anxiety?

Lesson 5

Learning About Perceived Exertion

Each student learns that the correct aerobic pace is determined by keeping his heart rate in the target heart rate zone. Sometimes, an individual must vary the pace to be correct because of stress, heat, humidity, wind, cold, and so on. This lesson teaches students to use heart rate monitors to stay alert, noticing if on different days or with different conditions their pace has to be adjusted. The lesson focuses on using the Rating of Perceived Exertion (RPE) in tandem with heart rate knowledge.

Goals:

- To recognize that the intensity that is right to produce the heart rate in the target zone one day may not be the right intensity to produce the heart rate in the target zone the next day. The variables of heat, wind, stress, emotions (e.g., anger), cold, humidity, sickness, overtraining, and so on may cause dramatic changes in heart rate response to the same exercise intensity.
- To learn to make adjustments accordingly, using heart rate to determine day-to-day exercise pace (intensity).

Key Concepts:

Heart rate monitors can provide authentic documentation of rating of perceived exertion (RPE) at the end of each unit of instruction. RPE refers to a person's subjective assessment (on a scale of 1 through 10) of how hard he or she is working (see table 6.2). Specifically, students will use heart rate data throughout the unit to learn to recognize the intensity that keeps them in their own target heart rate zones. At the end of the unit, students will demonstrate the ability to hold their heart rates in the correct target zone for 10 minutes—without continuous heart rate feedback—using the Polar Accurex II Heart Rate Monitor

with alarms turned off and the faces of the heart rate monitors concealed by wristbands or tape.

Materials:

- One heart rate monitor (such as the Polar Accurex II Heart Rate Monitor) for each student
- Masking tape or wristbands

Activity:

1. Have each student wear a heart rate monitor with her target heart rate zone programmed into the monitor (see chapter 3, lesson 2 for determining target heart rate zones). Remind students that when they are in their target heart rate zones, no alarms beep. But when the heart rate goes either too high or too low, according to an individual's target zone, the alarms beep, signaling the student to change the pace or intensity during the aerobic segment of class.

2. If using the Polar Accurex II Heart Rate Monitor, after each class period, have squad leaders record the following information on a chart for each student in their squads:
   - Average heart rate throughout class
   - Number of minutes in the target zone
   - Number of minutes below the target zone
   - Number of minutes above the target zone

If using the Polar Vantage XL Heart Rate Monitor, have squad leaders download and print out results.

3. Every quarter, give a final test to determine if each student has learned how to use perceived exertion. To conduct the test, assign students heart rate monitors for which you

have turned off the target zone alarms and covered the faces with masking tape. Thus, while the student's heart is being monitored he will not know its rate, forcing him to use ratings of perceived exertion to determine his correct pace during the aerobic segment of the class.

4. Have students begin the aerobic segment of the class. Tell them that they must hold their heart rates in the correct target zone to receive credit. Table 6.3 suggests grades based on the percentage of time spent keeping heart rate in target zone for the aerobic part of class.

TABLE 6.2   Borg Scale (Rate of Perceived Exertion)

0	Nothing at all
0.5	Extremely weak (just noticeable)
1	Very weak
2	Weak (light)
3	Moderate
4	
5	Strong (heavy)
6	
7	Very strong
8	
9	
10	Extremely strong (almost maximal)
•	Maximal

Teaching Tips:

Using the heart rate monitors, another easy method for scoring is to administer a 10-minute aerobic testing segment, scoring according to minutes in the target zone (table 6.4).

TABLE 6.3   Suggested Grades Based on Percent of Time

Percent of time heart rate held in target zone	Grade
90 to 100	A
80 to 89	B
70 to 79	C
60 to 69	D
below 59	F

TABLE 6.4   Suggested Grades Based on Minutes

Minutes in the target zone	Grade
9:00 to 10:00	A
8:00 to 8:59	B
7:00 to 7:59	C
6:00 to 6:59	D
5:59 or below	F

Notes

Lesson 6

Work, Stress, and Heart Rates

Students will find that many jobs or lifestyles that require or cause high heart rates throughout the day may or may not be physical in nature. Heart rates can reflect high stress, anger, or jobs that do not suit the individual (e.g., jobs that have high noise for those who truly dislike noise, indoor jobs for those who like the outdoors, and so on). Cardiovascular fitness is just as important for the individual who is at a desk all day as it is for the person who works physically hard on the job. The heart must be ready for extremes throughout life. If you have to run to catch a subway, run across the street through traffic, or be ready for an emotionally trying situation, your cardiovascular condition will be tested.

Goals:

- To encourage students to question the lifestyles they plan to lead, analyzing suitability.
- To learn what type of job situations may be suitable matches for their own interests, leading to healthier heart rates throughout the work day.

Key Concept:

We can record heart rates throughout the day, providing insight into various job situations and how the individual is handling the job.

Materials:

- One heart rate monitor with downloading capabilities (such as the Polar Vantage XL Heart Rate Monitor) for each student
- Computer access
- One worksheet 6.4 for each student

Activity:

1. Group students into five or six "heart rate teams."

2. Each team chooses a parent of one of the team members to wear a heart rate monitor for an entire workday. Teams should choose a back-up parent in case the first parent does not wish to participate.
3. Students check out a heart rate monitor the day before the parent is to wear it. Students show the parent how to operate the monitor and ask the parent to press the "recall" button several times throughout the workday, such as morning break, lunch, afternoon break, and end of workday.
4. After each parent has recorded his or her heart rate for one day, students bring back the monitor and download the information.
5. All students are given copies of each printout to analyze against each participant parent's job description, and are asked to discuss the following questions:

   - What was the average heart rate throughout the workday for each parent participant?
   - What was the highest heart rate throughout the workday for each parent participant?
   - Does overall cardiovascular conditioning for an individual affect these results, regardless of the type of job?
   - What does the heart rate throughout the day tell you about certain jobs?

Teaching Tips:

Review the graphs on worksheet 6.4 with students. Say "Notice that on one of the graphs, the heart rate was relatively low throughout the day except for one or two extremes. The other graph shows heart rates that are higher for longer periods of time."

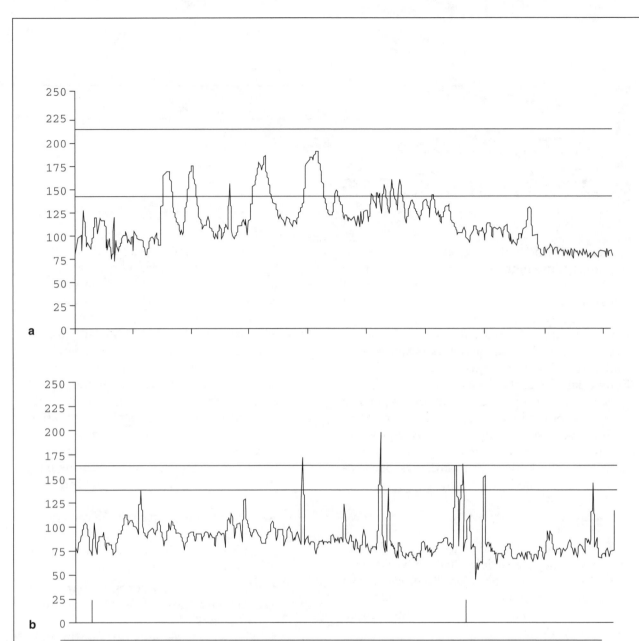

Figure 6.2 Two adults' heart rate graphs throughout the work day.

1. In the graphs of adults and their heart rates throughout the work day (figure 6.2, a and b), what types of jobs might cause you to have higher heart rates throughout the day and what types of jobs might allow you to have low heart rates throughout the day?

(continued)

2. One of these is a graph that shows an individual doing a job at a desk all day. The other is showing a graph of the heart rate of an individual who is working outside for certain periods of time. Which graph is which?

3. In either job, is it important to have good cardiovascular fitness? Why or why not?

4. If you elevate your heart rate only when you run across the street or when you experience stress in your job, do you need to have good cardiovascular fitness?

5. Do you think most adults pay attention to their heart rates throughout the day? Why or why not?

6. With heart disease costing this country $132 billion each year, what can you do to prevent heart disease?

Lesson 7

Faculty to Students—Getting to the Heart of Learning

Physical activity or increased heart rates don't always happen just in physical education class or during workouts or sports practices.

Goal:

- To see that while students and teachers are really in the same environment throughout the school day, their heart rates are a personal reminder of how the stresses and activities of the day are affecting them.

Key Concepts:

Heart rate data can add detail to our view of a school day, providing insight into the activity patterns or lack of activity patterns of both students and teachers (figure 6.3). While a school day may be exhausting for both, it may not be aerobic for either. That is why it is important to set aside time each day for aerobic conditioning. While certain times in a day may require excel-

lent cardiovascular conditioning, the typical day does not develop this conditioning—not without setting aside a workout time. Students should see that many teachers are standing, moving, and active throughout the school day, while many students are sedentary.

Materials:

- 20 heart rate monitors with downloading capabilities (such as the Polar Vantage XL Heart Rate Monitor)
- Computer access

Activity

1. Select 10 students and 10 faculty members to wear heart rate monitors throughout the same school day.
2. Have the students average the heartbeat totals for each group. Have them record who had the highest and lowest heartbeat

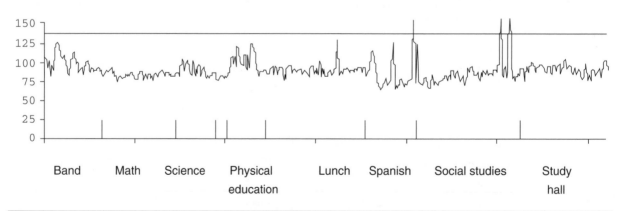

Figure 6.3   This student's heart rate fluctuated throughout the school day.

totals. Have the students discuss three reasons why.

3. Have the students compare the graphs for each group. Did some faculty have higher heartbeat totals than some students? Ask the students to tell you how their data reflect the teachers' and students' school days.

4. Ask the students: "Does stress affect the heart rate? Does age affect heart rates and the analysis of results? Is this apparent in the printout?"

Teaching Tips:

You can also try this lesson using heart rate monitors to record the heart rates of five boys and five girls during each class throughout the school day by having the student press the store/recall button at the beginning and ending of each class.

When you give the printouts back to the students, have each student write which class he or she was taking at each of the markings on the graph (when the store/recall button was pushed). Then, have each student figure out his or her average heart rate, highest and lowest heart rates, and heartbeat totals for the experiment.

Ask the students the following questions:

Was there a difference between the boys' and the girls' heart rate averages? Why or why not?

Does it appear that students are experiencing active school days or inactive school days?

What could be done to bring more activity into the school day?

How could the entire school benefit with an increase in activity time built into each school day?

What could the benefits be nationwide?

Notes

Lesson 8
24-Hour Heart Rate Log

Goals:

- To encourage students to focus on the time they spend doing specific activities each day.
- To encourage students to take control of their lifestyles and plan their days, rather than letting the day simply happen. (This is a problem for adults, too!)

Key Concepts:

A typical school day is sedentary, sitting at desks. Students must set aside time for exercise and relaxation, concentrating more on how to enjoy all aspects of the day.

Materials:

- One heart rate monitor with downloading capabilities (such as the Polar Vantage XL Heart Rate Monitor) for each student
- Computer access

Activity:

1. Have each student prepare a log detailing daily activities such as the following:

   7:00 A.M. Wake up
   7:15 Shower
   7:30 Get dressed
   7:45 Breakfast
   8:00 Arrive at school
   8:00 to 3:30 School schedule

4:00 After-school activities
6:00 Arrive home
6:30 Eat dinner
7:00 Study
9:00 TV and snack
10:00 Shower
10:30 Sleep

2. Have each student wear a heart rate monitor for one entire school day (or, if possible, before and after school, as shown on the sample schedule). Each student should push the store/recall button for major activities throughout the day.
3. Have students record their heart rates each hour next to their own written schedule of their own activities.
4. Ask students how daily routines are established. How or when do they make changes, and does scheduling time for specific needs work? Then have the students write their heart rates at the major markings in the log from the printout data for one day. Then have them evaluate their daily plans.

Teaching Tips:

If possible and with permission of students compare the daily logs of students who work, who work at home, who have to walk to school, and so on with those who do not work, do not walk to school, and so on. Speculate on the lifestyles of farmers versus town kids.

Lesson 9

Heart Rate and Weather

Try this activity on a hot and humid day to highlight the need to take weather into account when exercising. Be careful, though, to review the signs of heat stress, preventing dangerous situations.

using a heart rate monitor, however, the response can be controlled to remain at safe and consistent levels no matter what the temperature or weather.

Goal:

- To understand that heart rate is affected by the weather and that the response to exercise varies considerably because of this. By

Key Concepts:

Students can learn the various heart rate responses to weather by analyzing the data from a heart rate monitor.

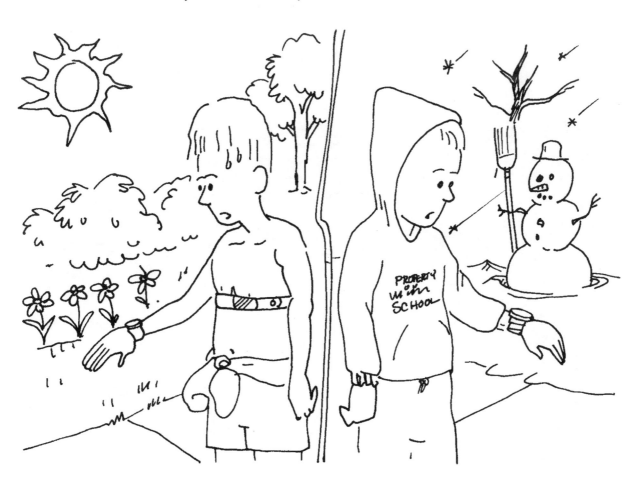

Materials:

- One heart rate monitor with downloading capabilities for each student
- One worksheet 6.5 for each student
- Computer access

Activity:

1. Break the students into five groups and assign each group to one of five practicing sport teams at the school (football, basketball, softball, swimming, soccer, cross-country, track, or the like).
2. Have each member of each group take a heart rate monitor to the team practice of the assigned sport and monitor one team member at that practice.

3. Have each group member download the team member's data and bring the print-out to class.

Teaching Tips

Be sure to get the coaches' permissions to allow the physical education class members to record their athletes' heart rates using the heart rate monitors.

Since worksheet 6.5 is long, you may decide to choose only particular questions from the list. Or, you can select one or two numbered sections on the list for the first class and the remaining questions for the following day. Thus, the assignment would be more manageable for both student and teacher.

Notes

1. Attach a printout from a heart rate monitor such as the Polar Vantage XL Heart Rate Monitor of your heart rate when the weather was hot and humid.

   - What happens to the heart rate when you exercise in hot and humid weather?

   - What are some risk factors of exercising in the heat and humidity if heart rate information is not constant and immediate?

   - What are some benefits of knowing your heart rate throughout exercise?

   - Do you think there are differences in heart rates of football players who have their helmets on during a hot and humid day while performing conditioning drills and those who do not?

   - If so, why?

   - Should coaches know the heart rates of their players during practices—especially on hot and humid days?

   - What about coaches of other sports: soccer, cross-country, running, baseball, soft-ball, or basketball?

   - How can athletes become conditioned to exercise safely when temperatures are high?

   - Name one way that conditioning could occur on hot and humid days in a way that would keep temperatures from artificially affecting heart rate.

(continued)

Worksheet 6.5

2. Compare the heart rates taken from the five different practices.
   • Which practice had the highest percentrage of time in the target zone?

   • Which printout had the highest heart rates?

   • Which printout had the lowest heart rates?

   • Which printout had the least amount of time in the target zone?

   • What are some reasons heart rates could vary throughout practice?

   • Do coaches know how any one practice affects any one player?

   • What could offer a solution for coaches?

3. Wear a heart rate monitor and run early in the morning for a definite distance. Wear a heart rate monitor and run the same distance after school.
   • Was there a difference in your heart rate when you ran the same distances but at different times?

   • Do you think it was the time of day, the temperature, or the body's readiness to exercise that made the difference?

   • How might cold weather affect the heart rate?

4. Record your heart rate running into the wind and then running with the wind. Make sure the distances are the same.

   • How did the wind affect your heart rate?

   • When people jog, do you think they take into account how wind affects their heart rate?

   • Should they? Why or why not?

CHAPTER

7

Heart Rate Sports: Games for All Ages

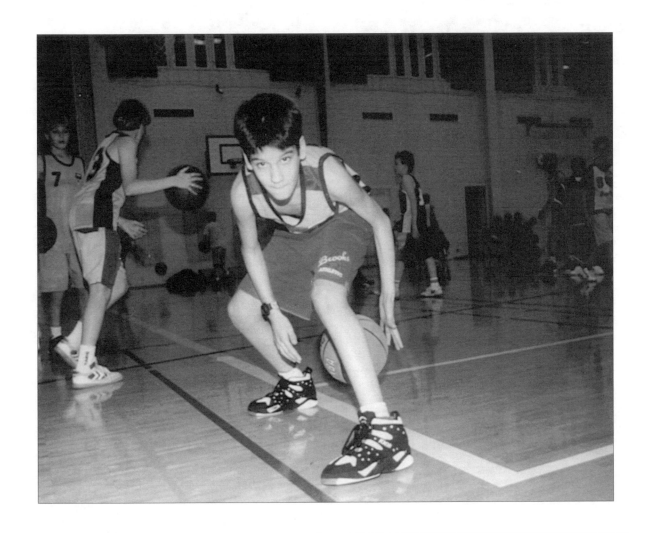

The games in this chapter use heart rates both to motivate and to assess, according to effort, individual performance in physical education throughout the school year. You can have students play these games, using the heart rate data they collect to create team or partner challenges.

We have designed the heart rate monitor sports described in this chapter to level the playing field through measuring effort in terms of heart rate, rather than student age, physical conditioning, talent, athletic ability, disabilities, gender, or race. By monitoring their heart rates, students take control of the effort outcome of the games. In-

deed, using heart rate monitors forces students to take personal responsibility for their efforts—an action that is likely to lead to a lifetime of fitness. In an age in which physical educators are struggling to apply the principles of authentic assessment, nothing could be more objective than measuring achievement in terms of heart rate minutes.

Use a variety of games to keep interest high throughout the year, correlating your choices to traditional units of study. Motivate students to focus on effort by helping them see that the common link among the games is the monitoring of heart rates.

Lesson 1

Heart Rate Flag Football

Play heart rate flag football, keeping track of heart rate energy to give credit for effort according to heart rate monitor data.

Goals:

- To recognize that heart rates will count throughout the class period and that effort (as measured by heart rate monitors) will especially count, actually contributing to the final score.
- To accept personal responsibility to make an all-out effort throughout class because effort will count toward the final outcome of the game.

Key Concepts:

No matter what activity is taking place in physical education class, you and your students should always measure effort. You should ask your stu-

dents to do their best throughout the school year. The heart rates will reflect the effort.

Materials:

- One football for each pair of teams
- One heart rate monitor (such as the Polar Accurex II) for each student
- Flags
- Football field

Activity:

1. Divide students into four-on-four flag football teams.
2. Have the modified games run the width of the field, using two of the 10-yard lines as the width of each modified game field.
3. Have each student wear a heart rate monitor and start recording at the beginning of the activity portion of class.

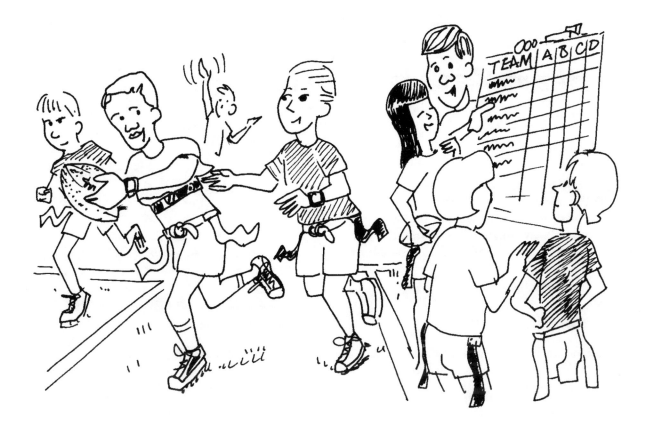

4. After the game, calculate the score for each team along the following parameters:

   - Record 10 yards gained for each minute a team member held her heart rate in the target zone.
   - Record 10 yards lost for each minute a team member was below their target zone.
   - Record a 10-yard penalty for each team member whose average heart rate fell below 130 beats per minute.
   - Score six points for each 100 yards gained by the team.
   - Score three points for each 50 yards gained by the team.
   - Score one extra point for each team member whose average heart rate was 140 beats per minute or above.

   - Add the actual game score for each team to their team heart rate score to arrive at the total score.

Teaching Tips:

Applying these rules, challenge other teams to see how many teams a particular team defeated—even though the team did not play them on that day. Hearts can win the game! Set up challenge teams between different physical education classes using the heart rate data. Or create challenges between homerooms, girls and boys, teachers and students, and so on. Using heart rate scoring allows all members of the team to be able to contribute equally and cooperatively.

Notes

Lesson 2
Heart Rate Basketball

Goals:

- To know that heart rates will count toward the win-loss record of each team.
- To recognize that we can measure effort using heart rates to help determine win-loss records, thereby allowing those who try hard, despite a lack of skill, to contribute as much as gifted athletes.

Key Concepts:

Similar to heart rate football, for this game, you give students credit for working at their personal bests, counting credit on the win-loss record of the team.

Materials:

- One heart rate monitor (such as the Polar Accurex II Heart Rate Monitor) for each student
- Basketballs
- As many courts as necessary for three- to five-player teams

Activity:

1. Divide students into three- to five-player teams, according to the facilities you have and the number and needs of your students.
2. Have students start their heart rate monitors when the basketball games begin.
3. After playing, determine the ultimate winner by adding the total combined target zone minutes of the team members plus minutes above the target zone (see table 7.1).

Teaching Tips:

Try the basketball format with volleyball or soccer games.

TABLE 7.1   Sample Calculations for Heart Rate Basketball

Red team: 35 points			Blue team: 34 points		
Name	Min. in target zone	Min. above target zone	Name	Min. in target zone	Min. above target zone
Kirk T.	22	4	Fred P.	20	3
Beth K.	20	2	Mary L.	19	1
Sara R.	23	1	Jane D.	24	3
Jason D.	19	4	Joshua K.	15	5
Dan W.	5	1	Joseph G.	13	0
	89 + 12 + 35 = 136			91 + 12 + 34 = 137	

Final score: Red 136
                    Blue 137

Lesson 3

Heart Rate Tennis

Goals:

- To use heart rate data to help determine players' intensity of play.
- To help to project to students that staying active is their responsibility.

Key Concepts:

Students are continuously moving throughout the class time, using heart rate data as the method for exchanging drill members with game members.

Materials:

- One heart rate monitor (such as the Polar Accurex II Heart Rate Monitor) for each student
- Tennis courts
- Tennis racquets and balls

Activity:

1. Assign two students to each court, one student on each side. Have these pairs each begin a game of singles tennis. Off each

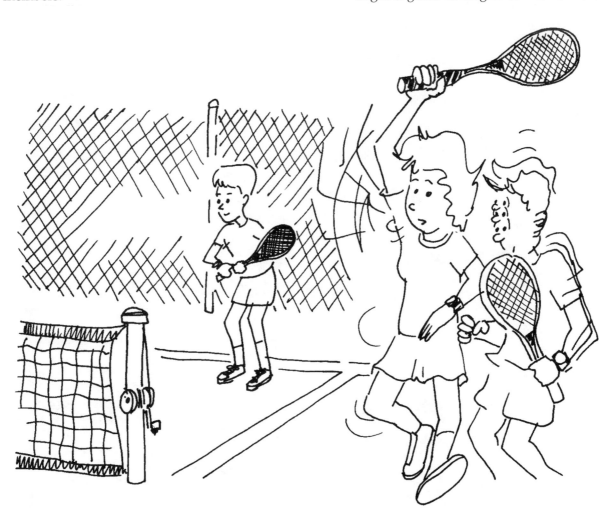

court, have one student stand at each end, ready to enter the game. These waiting students can dribble tennis balls until it is their turn to play.

2. Students playing the game continue to play until their heart rate drops out of their target zone as signaled by the beeping of the heart rate monitor. Whenever a student's monitor begins beeping, the waiting student replaces him on the court.

3. Remind students that their goal should be to see how little time they can spend outside the target zone and how much time can be spent inside the target zone.

4. Suggest that students can work at staying in the target zone by jumping up and down while waiting for an opponent to serve, by

running after loose balls, or by keeping the game going more steadily, all of which reduce time spent standing around.

5. Record the total time spent in, above, and below the target zone as well as the average heart rate of the physical education class for each student. The final score includes the total minutes in the target zone plus regular tennis scoring.

6. Each day, rotate students to different games.

Teaching Tips:

Ask "Did the game participants make a difference, or did the effort and energy of the student make the difference in who kept their heart rate in the target zone the most minutes?"

Notes

Lesson 4

Heart Rate Golf

Here's another fun way for students to chart individual heart rate target zone progress.

Goal:

- To use a golf course gameboard to move a "golf bag," which contains golf clubs that hit a golf ball various distances, according to minutes in the target zone, moving throughout the course, scoring pars, birdies, or bogeys each day.

Key Concepts:

When a golfer scores one less than the hole generally requires a good golfer to score, such as a score of three on a par four hole, this is called a birdie. Two hits less than par gives the golfer an eagle; three less is a double eagle. Students will score their "hits," using minutes in the target zone to see how they score using golfers' scorecards. As in golf, the student will be rewarded for achieving a great "hit" (minutes in the target zone beyond 10 minutes, in this case, 20 minutes) by getting to skip a space on the scorecard and move through the course at a faster pace. Different lengths of time in the target zone determine birdies, eagles, and double eagles—even holes-in-one! Students can use their scorecards to challenge other students to a "round" of golf (every nine weeks).

Materials:

- One scorecard for each student
- One heart rate monitor for each student

Activity:

1. Using the game board on page 106, have students move their "golf bags" one 10 TZ (target zone) space each time they hold their heart rates in the target zone for 10 minutes during physical education class.
2. As you read through the scoring (explained in step three), notice how a player has to earn either three, four, or five spaces to get to the next hole, according to whether the hole is a par three, four, or five.
3. If a student holds his heart rate in the target zone for 20 minutes in one physical education class, move two spaces as well as skip one extra space for a total move in one day of three spaces. If the student is on a par three hole, record the score as a hole-in-one! If the student is on a par four hole and records 10 minutes in the target zone the following physical education class, the student will have finished the hole in two "tries" (physical education class periods) and may record the score for the hole as an eagle—two under par. If the student is on a par five hole, and he moved three spaces one day and two spaces the next day, record a double eagle (three under par) because he finished the hole in two tries!
4. If a student fails to hold his heart rate in the target zone for at least 10 minutes, score an extra stroke for the hole, bogeying the hole.

Teaching Tips

If you use a par 36 golf course in physical education classes that meet twice a week, it will typically take one semester to complete the course: 36 class periods averaging 10 minutes in the target zone each physical education class period. Have students see how long it takes to "par" the course or how low a score each student can record using the extra space rule for 20 minutes or more in the target zone. To vary the game, you can change the par for every hole to 3. This set-up will take less time to complete.

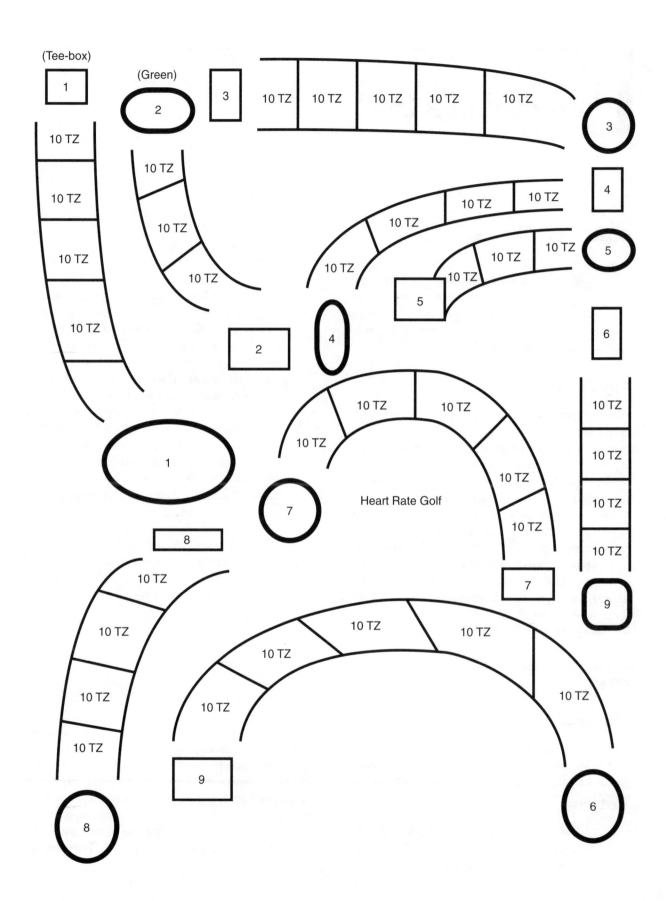

Heart Rate Golf

Lesson 5

Polar Baseball™

This activity offers a fun way to chart each student's fitness.

Goals:

- To elicit a personal best from each student in a competition made equitable by using heart rate data.
- To make heart rate monitoring fun in both team and individual efforts.
- To promote individual physical activity, teach perceived exertion, and improve self-esteem.

Key Concepts:

Polar Baseball™ is played without a bat or a ball, though conventional rules of hits and outs are followed. Students will receive credit for taking personal responsibility for keeping their heart rates in the correct target zone throughout class (see page 108). You can use the totals in friendly competitions, squad versus squad, class versus class, school versus school, state versus state, or even country versus country! No student is left out and all students can receive maximum credit for their efforts each day.

Players participating in a number of physical activities such as basketball, walking, jumping rope, or playing Frisbee can all be teammates. Since each participant is scored against her or his personal cardiovascular capabilities, the time spent in the predetermined heart rate zone, teams can also be made up of players of differing fitness levels. Physically challenged players can challenge the more physically abled; younger students can challenge older participants.

Materials:

- One heart rate monitor for each team member

- Blank Polar Baseball™ score card (see blank sample on page 109)

Activity:

1. The target heart rate zones of each participant are preset. Team lineup is posted prior to start of each game and cannot be changed until the game is finished. There are ten players to a team (number can be changed if other team agrees).
2. A Polar baseball game consists of three 30-minute innings (periods) played on three different days.
3. Athletes select the activity in which they wish to participate and monitor their heart rate while engaged in this activity. Each athlete's time in the target zone is automatically stored within the heart rate monitor and displayed on the receiver face when the exercise period is completed.
4. Innings end with three outs or once through the lineup, whichever comes first. Runners left on base at the end of an inning are stranded.
5. At the end of each inning, the information from the heart rate monitor is recorded on the scorecard. See completed sample scorecard on page 110. Like in baseball, the first batter up in the second inning is the batter that was scheduled to be up after the last batter in the first inning. As a reminder, at the end of each inning, draw a horizontal line in the next inning's column to indicate the lead-off batter for the next inning.
6. Each student's time in the target zone (tz) is then converted to hits and outs based on the following scale:

Target zone time	Baseball scoring
< 10:00	Out
10:00-11:59	Single
12:00-13:59	Double
14:00-14:59	Triple
15:00 or more	Home run

7. The winning team is the team that scores the most runs in three innings.
8. If a Polar Baseball™ league has been established, each team plays the same number of league games.

Teaching Tips:

Establish team lineups and have the students challenge one another, squads, or homerooms to see who wins the Polar Baseball tournament. Use the scorecard to determine the total score and the winners by adding "hits," which are the number of minutes in the target zone for that physical education period (inning). Allow students to challenge a different team to a baseball game every nine days.

At the end of the season (school term) playoffs and a world series can be played if enough teams participate. During these series games, the students can wear the heart rate monitor "blind"; that is, they will rely on perceived exertion and knowing whether or not they are working within their target heart rate zones, rather than relying on a beep from the monitor to tell them they are exercising at the right intensity.

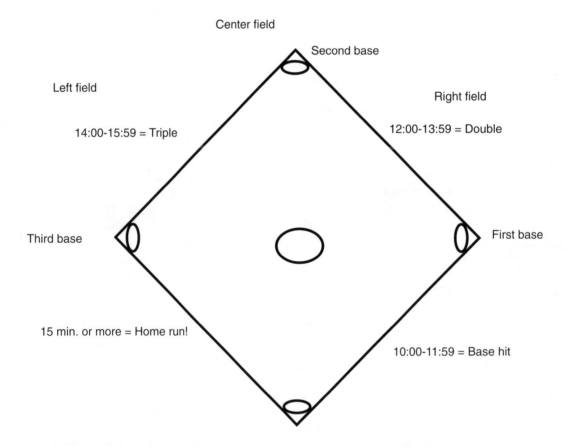

Center field

Second base

Left field

Right field

14:00-15:59 = Triple

12:00-13:59 = Double

Third base

First base

15 min. or more = Home run!

10:00-11:59 = Base hit

Sample Polar Scorecard

Name	Inning:		Date:			Inning:		Date:			Inning:		Date:		
	BaseRnrs	TZtime	Hit	Runs	Outs	BaseRnrs	TZtime	Hit	Runs	Outs	BaseRnrs	TZtime	Hit	Runs	Outs
		Total:					Total:					Total:			

Game Totals:

Polar Scorecard

ABC Middle School Team 3

Name	Inning: 1 Date: 8/2/96					Inning: 2 Date: 8/5/96					Inning: 3 Date: 8/7/96				
	BaseRnrs	TZtime	Hit	Runs	Outs	BaseRnrs	TZtime	Hit	Runs	Outs	BaseRnrs	TZtime	Hit	Runs	Outs
Andy	◇	12 10	D	—	—	◇	11 22	S			◇	9 50	O		1
Sasha	◇	14 17	T	1	—	◇	15 40	H	2		◇	10 12	S		
Min	◇	10 14	S	1	—	◇	12 19	D	—		◇	14 58	T	2	
Ollie	◇	9 58	—	—	1	◇	10 49	S	—		◇	9 33			1
Judy	◇	11 14	S	—	—	◇	13 01	D	1		◇				
Anne	◇	9 40	—	—	1	◇	15 01	H	3		◇				
Tony	◇	14 45	T	2	1	◇	12 02	D			◇				
John	◇	8 23				◇	10 12	S	1		◇				
Robert	◇					◇	15 10	H	1		◇	10 15	S		
Kim	◇					◇	7 14	—	—	1	◇	9 40	O		1
	Total:			4	3	Total:			7	1	Total:			2	3

Game Totals: 12 Runs

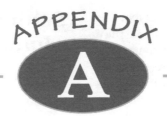

APPENDIX

A

Polar
Quick Instructions

Putting On the Heart Rate Monitor

1. With the wristwatch receiver on your wrist, place the chest belt high under your breasts with "Polar" right side up and as tight as comfortable.
2. Grasp the center of the belt transmitter; pull it away from your chest and wet the electrodes with either saliva, saline solution, or water. Release the transmitter and let it rest on your chest.

Operating Instructions

When HI/LO alarms have been set and the wristwatch is displaying the time do the following:

1. Press the red button once.

   The "♡" will start flashing with each heartbeat.

   The top display will begin counting time in minutes and seconds.

In approximately 5 to 10 seconds, your current heart rate will show in the bottom display.

To toggle the HI/LO alarms from on to off or from off to on, press the lower right button once; the "♡" appears when the alarm is active.

2. At the end of your exercise, press the upper right button once.

   The top display shows how long you've spent above the upper limit with a "♡."

   The bottom display shows your average heart rate for the workout.

   Press the red button once, and the time in the target zone will show in the upper display with the "TZ" symbol.

   Press the red button once again and the time below target zone will show in the upper display with "♡."

3. Press the upper right button twice to return to the time of day.
4. You can record up to 44 lap interval times and corresponding heart rate information by depressing the red button repeatedly

during the exercise. If you use this feature, lap times will show on the upper display while elapsed time will show on center display. To recall lap time and corresponding heart rate when in step 2, press the left button once. Proceed to play back lap-by-lap times by depressing the red button repeatedly. Press the upper right button twice at any time to return to the time of day.

Setting the Heart Rate Monitor

To set the time of day and alarm time, refer to pages 11 through 14 of the instruction manual.

To set the HI/LO target zone alarms, refer to page 18 of the instruction manual.

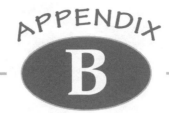

APPENDIX

B

NASPE Content Standards for Physical Education and Heart Rate Monitors

The National Association for Sport and Physical Education (NASPE) has released seven content standards that physical education programs should cover for all students. These seven outcome-based standards provide a basis for identifying individual program strengths and weaknesses and for setting realistic goals and strategies to align curriculum and instructional and assessment practices. Many of the lessons in this book apply these standards using Polar Heart Rate Monitors to authentically address and assess the individual learning.

1. **Student demonstrates competency in many movement forms and proficiency in a few movement forms.**

   See chapter 4, lesson 9.

2. **Student applies movement concepts and principles to the learning and development of motor skills.**

   See chapter 4, lesson 3.

   See chapter 4, lesson 9.

3. **Student exhibits a physically active lifestyle.**

   Heart rate monitors can be used to help students understand how active or inactive their lifestyle is and how heart rate is affected by anxiety, caffeine, stress, sleep.

   See chapter 4, lesson 4.

   See chapter 5, lesson 3.

   See chapter 6, lesson 6.

   See chapter 6, lesson 7.

   See chapter 6, lesson 8.

4. **Student achieves and maintains a health-enhancing level of physical fitness.**
   Using heart rate monitors, you can safely and accurately administer the mile-run or nine-minute run cardiovascular tests in the fall and again in the spring. You can place printouts from the tests in the students' portfolios, documenting the consistency of the students' efforts, thereby verifying the students' abilities to achieve cardiovascular

fitness as well as maintain or improve fitness throughout his or her school years. Specific information can be tracked that can signal future cardiovascular concerns.

See chapter 3, lesson 3.

See chapter 4, lesson 6.

See chapter 5, lesson 9.

5. **Student demonstrates responsible personal and social behavior in physical activity settings.**

Using heart rate monitors you can hold each student accountable for conducting themselves in a personally responsible manner through his own cardiovascular efforts throughout class.

See chapter 3, lesson 2.

See chapter 5, lesson 4.

6. **Student demonstrates understanding and respect for differences among people in physical activity settings.**

Using heart rate monitors a student will understand that cardiovascular conditioning is a personal experience and completely individual.

See chapter 5, lesson 1.

7. **Student understands that physical activity provides opportunities for enjoyment, challenge, self-expression, and social interaction.**

See all lessons!

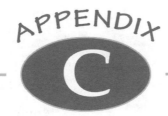
Funding Opportunities

I've had the privilege to spend the last 10 of my 20 years as a physical educator traveling across the United States and around the world speaking at conferences, advocating the infusion of technology into physical education to make the field more accountable and safe. Along the way, I have had the opportunity to look at many different ways to apply technology and have struggled—like many practitioners—to find ways to fund the purchase of the technology for my students' needs. With funding restrictions the norm in schools, physical education budgets have been reduced even as class sizes have increased! Concurrently, all other subject areas have adopted technological tools, using school funds established specifically for meeting the technological needs of the school district. Physical education, however, has been the last field of education to consider adding technology—largely because physical educators have not believed that these budgets included physical education.

Indeed, I have found that many of the physical educators in this country have no idea that most school districts have established technology committees. These committees seldom include physical educators as members, including only teachers of other subject areas and admin-istrators. This is a mistake! Since, however, each school district is free to establish their own system for dividing the funds for technology among their schools and teachers, I have discovered that most school districts require that teachers wanting to add technological tools to their classrooms must fill out a "Technology Application Form," describing the technology desired, the objectives for its use, the number of students who will be using it, the potential for the technology to perform as an assessment tool, the warranty provisions, where to purchase the technology, the cost per unit, who will train the teachers to use it, and so on.

When, after seeing a new technology in action, a physical educator becomes interested in it, the procedures for securing funding can overwhelm the teacher. With this in mind, I have developed these sample answers and have filled out a sample technology form to help guide you as you work to obtain what I believe is the most important of all technological tools available to physical education—the heart rate monitors. We believe that this form may be the most valuable funding tool available to the physical educator. It is our hope that these samples will inspire you to avail yourself of this technology.

—Beth Kirkpatrick

Summary of Heart Rate Monitor Uses in Public Education

Heart rate monitors can be gainfully used throughout the school district and from early morning into the evening and even on workdays. Coaches and staff can use the monitors at practices and in the classroom, and after school hours the monitors can be used in adult fitness classes.

Just think about the uses: The dream of all coaches and players is having access to equipment such as that used by professional athletes and Olympic stars to obtain maximum training effects from their efforts! When this same equipment can optimize training affects for long-distance runners; sprinters; football, basketball, hockey, and soccer players as well as almost all individual and team sport participants, this equipment becomes even more desirable. On learning that the equipment is moderately priced, can be used indoors or outdoors, on the field or in the water, in hot or cold weather *and* acts as a preprogrammed electronic coach that prompts, measures, and records an individual's training efforts, this equipment changes from desirable to essential. This dream piece of equipment is the heart rate monitor.

Heart rate monitors such as the Polar Vantage XL and Polar Accurex II HRMs have been used by Olympic stars throughout the world to obtain the cardiovascular edge as they trained to peak condition. Some professional football teams have even structured how they call plays based on the heart rate reserve of their players. Having used the heart rate monitors in practice and played back the results, coaches were able to predetermine which players' hearts had recovered, depending on the sequence of plays called.

In another example, high ranked college basketball teams found that their star players were not practicing at a high enough heart rate to prepare them for the last two minutes of a tough game. While using heart rate monitors, other coaches found that a good number of the athletes never recovered during interval training, resulting in a loss of training benefits. With this accurate information, these coaches were able to design more effective practices.

But we understand that you may need to be as efficient with your funds as your workouts. To maximize school purchases and still have full use of the coach's dream tool, the coaches and physical education teachers in your school can share the heart rate monitors, one department using them during the day, the other, after school.

Keep these uses in mind when you approach your school's technology committee with a funding request for heart rate monitors. It is a good idea to list many of the uses heart rate monitors can have for your classes and for the district as a whole. You may want to include a list of such uses (as those highlighted below) with your funding request.

Individual Programming During Physical Education Classes

- Programs correct aerobic pace for each student during aerobic segment of class.
- Reinforces knowledge of correct pace and identifies students with similar aerobic paces.
- Provides immediate feedback in the form of visualization of proper heart rate—a motivating factor.
- Reflects and records resting and recovery heart rates and time.
- Acknowledges weather factors and how they affect exercise (heat, cold, and wind).
- Diagrams effectiveness of use of class time by the student as well as the teacher.
- Safely projects progression rates in both distance and pace increases.

- Helps determine format and curriculum effects on each student.
- Provides evidence that alternate forms of aerobic conditioning create effects on the cardiovascular condition (e.g., rowing machines, ergometers, cross-country ski machines, ladder machines, stair steppers, rope jumping, swimming, and the like).
- Complements testing: heart rates determined more accurately; provides printout to enhance computations; lets more students test per session; gives input for individuals providing confidence in accuracy of the cardiovascular test; and monitors students during the test to prevent accidents, increasing safety.
- Provides fall to spring comparisons of target heart rates to allow progressions and shows you how to determine improvement according to the individual heart rate and intensity—not according to how a student can "gut it out."
- Monitors special needs children or children with specific health risks (high percent body fat, heart murmurs, high blood pressure, asthma, allergies.)

Class Usage

- Helps you objectively evaluate the subjective analysis—grading by comparing the subjective data with the printout.
- Helps you compare aerobic conditioning progression rates per class: males with females, athletes with nonathletes, elementary with middle schoolers, and middle schoolers with high schoolers.
- Provides data for accurate comparisons of individuals year to year.
- Helps you evaluate class format (e.g., flexibility drills throughout class rather than all at once.)

- Diagrams effectiveness of class time usage as well as curriculum benefits: which activities promote the most aerobic benefits, the most anaerobic, and so on.
- Highlights differences that affect conditioning: field size, activity space, size of a class, modified games compared to regulation, motivation benefits (when wearing heart rate monitor as compared to not—accountability)
- Helps you determine many other influences:
  1. The cycle of fitness or if there is one
  2. Climate
  3. Burn out evident or progression effective
  4. The similarities or differences within the same class involving the same activities on the same day
  5. The similarities or differences involving the same activities on the same day for different classes

Comparing Our Physical Education Program to Other Programs

- The elementary, middle school, and high school programs within the district
- Each interscholastic sport within the school
- Schools with students of comparable fitness and progress
- Schools that use similar programs and those that use entirely different programs
- Rural or suburban schools and inner-city schools
- State comparisons and climate comparisons
- Accountability of program and instructors, perhaps those with the same format, different instructors, and so on
- Curriculums of and formats used in other schools

Technology Committee Funding Request Form for Hardware and Software

State the Problem and Provide the Solution

Does the request meet the school-wide vision? (See pages 116 and 117 in this book for some ideas regarding the multiple uses of heart rate monitors.)

The Problem

Cardiovascular disease is the number one killer in America. Lack of exercise is considered to be one of the major risk factors for heart disease. Research shows that 90 percent of children who fail to exercise adequately in their teenage years also do not exercise adequately when they become adults.

Physical education is the only class that students take throughout their school years that is responsible for addressing and assessing cardiovascular fitness. In every battery of physical education tests that are traditionally given throughout the country, cardiovascular fitness assessments are included—whether it is the mile run or the 9- or 12-minute run. In all of these tests that are recommended by the President's Council on Physical Fitness; the American Association of Health, Physical Education, Recreation and Dance (AAHPERD); the National Association for Sport and Physical Education (NASPE); and the Cooper Aerobic Institute, however, heart rates are completely unknown for nearly every student in nearly every cardiovascular fitness test that is given in this country. Not only does this put every child at risk, it jeopardizes the accuracy of these tests. Without accurate knowledge of heart rate throughout the testing and throughout every activity each child participates in throughout their school years, it is no wonder that we have had generation after generation graduating without basic knowledge of heart health. Not only has their educational experience failed to teach them how to individualize exercise, it has perpetuated ignorance through false testing. Heart rates were never known throughout their education, therefore they perceive that heart rate must be unimportant when it comes to exercise and testing cardiovascular fitness. The result has been that in the United States, cardiovascular fitness continues to decline, percent body fat continues to increase, and risk factors for heart disease are now known to exist in nearly half of the elementary children in this country. It is no wonder that it is costing this country nearly $130 billion a year to treat cardiovascular disease!

The Solution

The Polar Vantage XL Heart Rate Monitor is now being used in thousands of schools nationwide. Using a wireless transmitter that is encased in a waterproof chest

(continued)

strap that houses two electrodes, the heart rate is accurately transmitted to a wristwatch-style heart rate monitor that continuously displays the heart rate throughout the time that the individual is wearing it. It can be programmed to signal the individual if the heart rate is either at unsafe or nonbeneficial levels for that individual. Once the exercise is completed, the heart rate monitor can interface with a computer and the student or teacher can download information and print out a hardcopy, showing the complete workout or testing heart rate graphically displayed and fully analyzed. Each heart rate monitor can store up to eight different files, allowing the teacher to use it all day before downloading it.

These heart rate monitors provide instant feedback, scientific information for individualizing student's workouts, motivation through accountability, safety in assessing and addressing cardiovascular fitness, portfolio data for each student, information to share with parents and students, curriculum design accountability, teacher accountability, a scientific tool for homework assignments, and interdisciplinary education through combining physical education with science and math.

Is the Technology Requested User-Friendly?

On a scale of "1" to "5" (with "1" being very easy and "5" being difficult) rank the following question: "How user-friendly is the requested technology?"

How Do You Know You Need It?

Without heart rate monitors, there is no possible way to know if any single student or class of students has safely and properly exercised in the appropriate heart rate zones necessary to achieve a training effect. Since no two students are alike, no scientific way to teach cardiovascular fitness exists without knowledge of heart rate. Moreover, no scientific way to test cardiovascular fitness without heart rate knowledge exists. Furthermore, without technology, the teacher cannot place a single printout in a student's portfolio to demonstrate either effort or accountability in physical education. Heart rate monitors have proven to be a success in thousands of schools in the United States. Students vary in sizes, medical conditions, percents body fat, fitness levels, and attention spans. Heart rate monitors are like personal fitness trainers that will alert students according to their heart rates at any time throughout the workout or testing situation. No one should be working without knowledge of heart rate. Technology has entered every facet of our lives. Now let it enter the quest to prevent heart disease and promote heart health in our children.

(continued)

Training and Dissemination of Information

How, when, and where are you going to communicate the purposes and uses of this request to the faculty? In the case of Polar Heart Rate Monitors, instructional videos accompany each purchase. Polar also can arrange an instructional workshop given by one of their consultants. In addition, Ball State University conducts heart rate monitor training workshops throughout the year. To set up a Polar Heart Rate Monitor Technology Workshop for your school, district, or area, contact Polar Electro, Inc., at 1-800-227-1314 (extension 3061 or 3021).

Sample Technology Request

Date requested: _____   Date reviewed: _____

Name: _____   Position: _____

Description of request: _____

_____

_____

_____

_____

Hardware/software (circle one)

Name of product: _____

Supplier information:

    Cost:

        For equipment _____   For shipping _____

        Other costs (maintenance, extra
        equipment, annual subscriptions
        or upgrades, etc.) _____

(continued)

Type of use (check one):

___ Instructional   ___ Management and record keeping

___ Drill and practice   ___ Communication and presentations

___ Simulation

User population:

___ Student   ___ Community   ___ School-wide

Breadth of use:

___ Individual classroom   ___ Department (list)   ___ Team (list)

___ School-wide

Estimated frequency of use:

___ Daily   ___ Weekly   ___ Other (describe):

_____

_____

_____

_____

Other details:

Sample Letter Explaining Polar HRMs to Parents

Dear Parents:

This year in physical education class all students will have the opportunity to use the heart rate monitors. These heart rate monitors provide immediate feedback for the student as well as the teacher. Continuous heart rate is recorded for each student wearing the combination heart rate monitor and electrode, which is encased in a chest strap. The invaluable information that each heart rate monitor provides affords each student the opportunity to learn to exercise according to individual level of conditioning. No two students are exactly alike in terms of physical conditioning. With the use of the heart rate monitors, our students will now be given credit for doing their personal bests and will be exercising according to what is safe for their level of conditioning. Heart rate summaries from each physical education class will be recorded for all students wearing the heart rate monitors and will be included in their portfolios. Students will now have the documented data that their efforts in physical education class do count and that exercise is truly an individual experience.

Because the heart rate monitors require the use of an electrode encased in a chest strap, which includes an elastic belt and transmitter, the repeated use of the elastic belt throughout the day for each class requires the constant adjustment of the strap by the instructor during the class and the cleansing of the strap throughout the day. This results in loss of class time and in extreme wear and tear on the elastic straps.

We would like to make available the option for all students to purchase their own personal elastic chest strap that would be preset for their own individual use. This also eliminates the constant between-class cleansing of the straps and the more efficient use of the instructor's time. Individual elastic straps give students a more personal involvement with the use of technology and the confidence that the elastic straps are more easily kept clean.

The cost of one elastic strap is $ _____. This one-time investment will mean your child does not have to share the elastic strap with anyone else throughout the school year. If you should decide that this is an option you would like to exercise, please send in $ _____ with your child.

Thank you for returning this form signed, and we look forward to an exciting school year using this new technology to bring safety, enjoyment, and an individualized approach to exercise. Stop in and we would be happy to demonstrate how the heart rate monitors work.

Yours in fitness and health,